OXFORD MEDICAL PUBLICATIONS

Oxford Handbook of

Rehabilitation Medicine

Oxford Handbooks

Oxford Handbook of
Rehabilitation Medicine

Michael P. Barnes

Professor of Neurological Rehabilitation
University of Newcastle upon Tyne,
Hunters Moor Regional Rehabilitation Centre,
Newcastle upon Tyne, UK

and

Anthony B. Ward

Consultant in Rehabilitation Medicine
University Hospital of North Staffordshire,
North Staffordshire Rehabilitation Centre,
Stoke on Trent, UK

OXFORD
UNIVERSITY PRESS

OXFORD
UNIVERSITY PRESS

Great Clarendon Street, Oxford OX2 6DP

Oxford University Press is a department of the University of Oxford.
It furthers the University's objective of excellence in research, scholarship,
and education by publishing worldwide in

Oxford New York

Auckland Bangkok Buenos Aires Cape Town Chennai
Dar es Salaam Delhi Hong Kong Istanbul Karachi Kolkata
Kuala Lumpur Madrid Melbourne Mexico City Mumbai Nairobi
São Paulo Shanghai Taipei Tokyo Toronto

Oxford is a registered trade mark of Oxford University Press
in the UK and in certain other countries

Published in the United States
by Oxford University Press Inc., New York

Formerly published as *Textbook of Rehabilitation Medicine* 2000
First published as an *Oxford Handbook* 2005

A catalogue record for this title is available from the British Library

ISBN 0 19 852896 5

10 9 8 7 6 5 4 3 2 1

Typeset by Newgen Imaging Systems (P) Ltd., Chennai, India.
Printed in Italy
on acid-free paper by Legoprint S.p.A

Preface

Rehabilitation Medicine is a relatively new and emerging specialty. It is now an integral part of most medical undergraduate curricula and has an increasingly important role in many postgraduate training programmes. There is now evidence that rehabilitation can produce real benefits for people with disabilities and for their carers. There are increasing numbers of stroke units and other rehabilitation facilities in many hospitals. Thus, many more medical practitioners and senior nursing and therapy staff will come into contact with rehabilitation services in the coming years.

This book is intended for a wide audience. First, we hope it is a useful and succinct summary of the field of rehabilitation for the medical student. However, we hope that the book will not be so confined, but will also be useful for junior doctors, therapists, nurses, and psychologists working in close conjunction with rehabilitation physicians. We also hope that it is informative, useful and, above all, imparts a sense of the real benefits that can accrue from an interdisciplinary rehabilitation programme.

Michael Barnes, Newcastle upon Tyne
Anthony Ward, Stoke on Trent
2004

Contents

21 Parkinson's disease and movement disorders

22 Motor neuron diseases

23 Disorders of the peripheral nerves

29 Ageing and disablity

Concepts of rehabilitation

Introduction

What are the basic concepts of rehabilitation medicine? In many ways rehabilitation is different from most other medical specialties. It is primarily a process of education of the disabled person so that, ideally, they can cope with family, friends, work, and leisure with as little support as possible. Thus, rehabilitation is a process that centrally involves the disabled person in making plans and setting goals that are important and relevant to their own circumstances. Rehabilitation is not a process that is done *to* the disabled person but it is a process that is done *by* the disabled person with the guidance, support, and help of a wide range of professionals as well as family and friends. Rehabilitation is also a process that goes beyond the rather narrow confines of physical disease and also deals with the psychological consequences of disability as well as the social milieu in which the disabled person has to function. A key factor that differentiates rehabilitation from most of medicine is that it is not a process that can be carried out by medical practitioners alone and of necessity requires the active partnership of a whole range of health and social service professionals. The characteristics of rehabilitation are shown in Table 1.1.

Table 1.1 Characteristics of rehabilitation

It is an educational process
Crucial involvement of the disabled person in programme planning
Key involvement of family, friends, and colleagues
It is a process that requires clear goals to be set and measured
It is a multidisciplinary process
It is a process based on the concepts of disability (activity) and handicap (participation)

Impairment, disability, and handicap

The key principles that lie behind rehabilitation are those that were proposed by the World Health Organization in 1980—impairment, disability, and handicap. These are fundamental to rehabilitation. Impairment is simply a descriptive term that says nothing about consequence. A right hemiparesis, for example, or a left-sided sensory loss, or a homonymous hemianopia are impairments. However, the right hemiparesis can be relatively mild leading to virtually no functional consequence or can be profound leading to complete inability to walk. It is the functional consequence of the impairment that is described as the disability. Rehabilitation goes beyond impairment and looks at the functional context and tries to minimize the impact of the disability. It is, after all, the disability that matters to the individual and not the impairment. Rehabilitation medicine does not minimize the importance of diagnosis and impairment in an effort to understand the underlying pathophysiology but simply places equal emphasis on the consequent disability.

Handicap goes one step further. Handicap describes the social context of the disability. In our example of a right hemiparesis even a relatively mild right-sided weakness can have profound implications for a young man who is a scaffolder or who wanted to go into the armed services as such occupations would be closed to him or an existing job may be lost. However, an older man who is already retired and whose abilities are restricted by other problems such a disability may have limited impact on his lifestyle. Handicap does not only deal with the broader physical consequence of a disability but looks at the broader social context. A mild hemiparesis, for example, in a receptionist may not actually prevent that person from undertaking the job and being a good employee. However, the attitude of the employer to the disabled person may cause her to be moved elsewhere or even lose her job. A person who needs to use a wheelchair may be quite capable of undertaking their job but cannot access the office because it is not wheelchair accessible. Rehabilitation needs to take into account not only the disability but also the particular handicap for that person and thus rehabilitation strays into the arena of societal attitudes and the physical environment, which are traditionally outside the realm of medicine.

Recently the World Health Organization has produced a new classification, which has less negative connotations. Disability is now termed *activity* and handicap is now termed *participation*. This classification works on the same principles but obviously places more emphasis on the individual's abilities rather than disabilities and on the social context of the disability (Table 1.2).

Table 1.2(a) Definitions of the World Health Organization's International Classification of Impairments, Disabilities, and Handicaps (1980)

Impairment: any loss or abnormality of psychological, physiological, or anatomical structure or function

Disability: any restriction or lack of activity resulting from an impairment to perform an activity in the manner or in the range considered normal for people of the same age, sex, and culture

Handicap: a disadvantage for a given individual resulting from impairment or disability that limits or prevents the fulfilment of a role that would otherwise be normal for that individual

Table 1.2(b) New classifications of the International Classification of Function and Disability (ICIDH II)

Impairment: loss or abnormality of a body structure or of a physiological or psychological function

Activity: the nature and extent of functioning at the level of the person. Activities may be limited in nature, duration, and quality

Contextual factors: include the features, aspects, and attributes of objects, structures, (participation) human-made organizations, service provision, and agencies in the physical, social, and attitudinal environment in which the people live and conduct their lives. Contextual factors include both environmental factors and personal factors

After Halbertsma, J., Heerkens, Y.F., Hirs, W.M. (2000). Towards a new ICIDH: International Classifications of Impairments, Disabilities and Handicaps. *Disability and Rehabilitation* **22**, 144–56.

Medical model of disability

The new classification of impairment, activity, and participation is a step towards a social model of disability and a step away from the medical model of disability. These terms are in common usage in the field of rehabilitation and need further description. The medical specialty of rehabilitation medicine has come from an 'illness' background. It has in the past been a specialism that in general has been carried out by physicians with the support of nurses and therapists and delivered to disabled people. This health-related and illness-related perspective of disability is known as the medical model of disability. It assumes several things about the nature of disability (Table 1.3).

The philosophy of medicine has traditionally been to treat and to cure but in rehabilitation these outcomes are unlikely and the aim has been to normalize. This philosophy was reinforced by the initial classification of the World Health Organization that produced a distinction between impairment, disability, and handicap. The medical model of disability usually implies that it is the physician who should take a leading role in the entire rehabilitation process—being team leader, organizing programmes of care, and generally directing the delivery of services for the disabled person. The doctor/patient relationship was the senior relationship in the medical model. Rehabilitation was born around the First World War when there was a very strong philosophy of the doctor telling injured servicemen how to behave, how to get better, and how to get back as quickly as possible to active duty. Such a model may have been appropriate in that cultural context but is now outdated. In recent years the central role of the physician has, in general, been subsumed by the central role of the multidisciplinary team. It is now realized that all health and social service professionals have their own role to play in the overall rehabilitation programme for the disabled person. However, even modern multidisciplinary rehabilitation is still largely based on the philosophy of the medical model—just a little watered down.

Table 1.3 Assumptions of the medical model of disability

Disability is individualized. It is regarded as a disease state that is located within an individual. Thus, the problem and solution may both be found within that person
Disability is a disease state. A deviation from the norm. It inherently necessitates some form of treatment or cure
Being disabled, a person is regarded inherently as biologically or psychologically inferior to that of the able-bodied and normal human being
Disability is viewed as a personal tragedy. It assumes the presence of a victim. The objective normality state that is assumed by professionals gives them a dominant decision-making role often noted in a typical doctor/patient relationship

After Laing, R. (1998). A critique of the disability movement. *Asia Pacific Disability and Rehabilitation Journal* **9**, 4–8.

Social model of disability

Disability lobby groups have long suggested that the fundamental construct of disability is that a person's impairment is not the cause of their restriction of activity but rather it is the organization of society that discriminates against them. The social model focuses on the fact that disability is a construction of society and if society could accept and accommodate disabled people, both physically and attitudinally, then disability as a concept would be made redundant. The key features of the social model are listed in Table 1.4.

As the disability movement developed, particularly in the United States after the Vietnam War and in the UK in the 1980s, there was a feeling of antagonism between health professionals involved in disability on the one hand and activists in the disability movement on the other hand. There was limited cooperation. These two extreme positions have now rather softened and disabled people realize that health professionals have a clear and important role in helping to minimize activity restrictions. This is particularly true in the post-acute setting after, for example, stroke or traumatic brain injury. Even in longer-term disability, such as cerebral palsy or multiple sclerosis, the health professional still has a key role to play. The crude dichotomy between the medical model and the social model is slowly but surely being replaced by a more appropriate halfway house—which could be called the *partnership model of disability*.

Table 1.4 Assumptions of the social model of disability

A person's impairment is not the cause of restriction of activity
The cause of restriction is the organization of society
Society discriminates against disabled people
Attitudinal, sensory, architectural, and economic barriers are of equal, if not greater, importance than health barriers
Less emphasis is placed on the involvement of health professionals in the life of the disabled person

Terminology

In the disability literature and in clinical practice it is vital to use correct terminology. This is not mere political correctness. Incorrect terminology can not only be demeaning but can indicate an inappropriate philosophy or attitude from the individual concerned or indeed from the whole multi-disciplinary team.

It is important to avoid terminology that implies dependency or terminology which just categorizes all disabled people. The word 'patient', for example, may be entirely appropriate for someone who is acutely ill and in the short term dependent upon medical and health professionals. However, in rehabilitation, if one agrees with the philosophy underlying the social model of disability, then disabled people are not ill and thus 'patient' is not a term that is appropriate. When the rehabilitation process is striving to give that person independence and develop new skills then terminology that implies the opposite should be avoided. There are a number of other group classifications that must be avoided including:

- epileptics
- stroke sufferers
- MS (multiple sclerosis) sufferers
- spastics
- young chronic sick
- the handicapped
- the disabled.

Although there is no universally accepted terminology it does seem reasonable to use the term 'disabled person' or 'person with a disability'. Correct terminology simply means that the person is being treated as an individual and not simply labelled as an example of a particular group.

As with many sections of society, it does seem acceptable for the group members themselves to use self-derogatory terms. People with spinal cord injuries will often refer to themselves as 'paras' or 'tetras' or even 'crips'.

Disability terminology is a minefield waiting to trap the unwary. The strength of feeling on these issues should not be underestimated.

Approaches to rehabilitation

Rehabilitation can be defined as an active and dynamic process by which a disabled person is helped to acquire knowledge and skills in order to maximize physical, psychological, and social function. It is a process that maximizes functional ability and minimizes disability and handicap—thus promoting activity and participation. There are three basic approaches in rehabilitation:

- Approaches to reduce disability.
- Approaches designed to acquire new skills and strategies, which will reduce the impact of the disability.
- Approaches that help to alter the environment, both the physical environment and the social environment, so that a given disability carries with it as little handicap as possible.

These are three vital concepts to the understanding of the rehabilitation process. The following is an example of these three approaches in action.

Case example

A middle-aged man has multiple sclerosis. He has been working quite successfully in the post room of a large factory. He is married with two children and has an active social life. However, in recent months he has developed increasing problems with walking secondary to developing paraparesis complicated by spasticity. In addition he has recently developed difficulties with urinary frequency and urgency. Rehabilitation, using our three basic approaches, could be structured as follows:

- Attempts could be made to reduce his disability by appropriate treatment of his spasticity and use of medication to control his bladder symptoms.
- He could learn new skills. He could learn, for example, to walk with external support such as a stick or even use a wheelchair for longer distances such as from the office car park to his place of work. He could be taught intermittent self-catheterization to assist his urinary problems.
- Approaches could be made to alter his work environment. He may, for example, be advised on the use of a perching stool so he can support himself whilst sorting the post. He may need to approach his employer to change or reduce his hours if prolonged periods of standing are leading to increasing fatigue. At home there may be a need to provide grab rails in the toilet or other adaptations to the bathroom or kitchen. His wife and family will clearly need to be involved in order to understand his condition and adjust the family lifestyle to cope with his new problems. His wife may begin to share the driving if problems of spasticity are beginning to interfere with his driving abilities over long distances.

Thus, there are many simple pointers that could help him to minimize the impact of his condition on his work, on his family, and on his leisure time. The rehabilitation team needs to keep in mind these three basic approaches when planning the rehabilitation programme.

Goal setting

The essence of rehabilitation is goal setting. The first goal to be established is the final strategic aim. This can vary significantly. For some a long-term goal would be returning to a completely normal lifestyle. For others it may simply be to return home and remain at home with the help of carers. In other cases it may be to take up part-time employment or resume a particular leisure interest. Sometimes much discussion, and even argument, is necessary in order that all parties can agree a realistic long-distance strategic goal. After such a goal has been established then steps need to be identified in order to achieve that goal. If, for example, a long-term goal is to be independently mobile without the use of aids then achieving that goal can be broken down into a number of shorter-term subgoals. This may, for example, start with sitting without support, then standing without support, then walking with assistance, then walking with aids, and finally independent walking over increasing distances. It is important to emphasize that the goals must be precise. It is inappropriate, for example, to set a goal such as to walk with an improved gait. This is not specific or measurable and is obviously open to considerable subjective interpretation. A better subgoal would be to walk 20 metres with the aid of a stick within a period of 30 seconds. Thus, goals need to be both specific and measurable. They also need to be achievable within the context of the underlying natural history or pathophysiology of the condition. In order for progress to be seen it is also useful for goals to be time limited. In a post-acute rehabilitation setting it is useful to plan for achievable subgoals in a period of 1 or perhaps 2 weeks whereas in people with longer-term disabilities such goals could be set over a much longer timescale. Finally each goal must be relevant for that individual. It may be relevant for some people to learn how to make a cup of tea but for others it may be more relevant to learn how to open a can of lager!

In summary, it is useful to remember the mnemonic SMART when goals are being met. All goals should be:

- **S**pecific
- **M**easurable
- **A**chievable
- **R**elevant
- **T**ime limited.

Outcome measurement

The disabled person and the rehabilitation team need to know when the goals have been achieved. It is important for each goal to have a valid and reliable outcome measure attached to it. A number of specific outcome measures are discussed later in this handbook. In summary, there are a number of measures that have been designed to monitor overall disability and/or quality of life that are useful for assessing progress towards longer-term goals. Shorter-term subgoals often need more specific outcome measures. Such examples would be specific measures of mobility, such as timed walking speed, specific measures of hand function, such as the Action Research Arm Test, or more specific psychological parameters, such as an objective measure of memory. Any outcome measure used needs to be specific to the outcome it is measuring as well as being both valid and reliable. There is little point in using an outcome measure that has not been validated and shown to be reliable for the particular circumstances in which it is used. This would be like measuring cooking ingredients on scales with the wrong weights. However, the scales need not, and indeed preferably should not, be complicated or time-consuming. Whilst specific and somewhat complicated measures of mobility are sometimes useful, particularly in a research setting, simple day-to-day, but objectively measurable goals, can also be used in a busy clinical situation. The ability to hold a saucepan with a give volume of water for a particular period of time is an example of a simple and objective goal that may be of practical relevance to that individual.

Whilst objectively measurable goals are useful it should obviously not be forgotten that the opinion of the disabled person and/or their family is of primary importance and should always be able to colour and adjust any objective measure. Objective measurement, whilst vital, should not be allowed to override the opinions, perceptions, and wishes of the disabled person. Indeed the disabled person should be the central figure in the setting of goals and their appropriate measurement and monitoring.

Benefits of rehabilitation

The specific benefits of rehabilitation will become self-evident in the later sections of this book. However, in general terms the benefits of rehabilitation can be summarized as follows:

• Functional benefit. There is now significant evidence that a coordinated interdisciplinary rehabilitation approach can produce better functional outcome than traditional unidisciplinary service delivery. In terms of stroke, for example, a rehabilitation unit will produce more functional gain, more quickly, with a better chance of returning home and with decreased morbidity and mortality. There is a similar case in the context of traumatic brain injury. There is even now evidence of a functional benefit of rehabilitation in deteriorating conditions, such as multiple sclerosis. These specific issues are discussed in later sections. There is also now evidence that short-term gains in a rehabilitation unit can generalize into longer-term functional improvements. If longer contact with the rehabilitation team is not established then the short-term functional gains and new skills may fade with time. This emphasizes the importance of not only post-acute rehabilitation units but also longer-term community support as well as rehabilitation support for those with deteriorating problems. What is not known is which elements of the rehabilitation process produce such functional benefits. Is it the basic rehabilitation process or is it simply the multidisciplinary or interdisciplinary team—or both combined. There is room for much more research on this subject but it is very likely that it is the whole rehabilitation process outlined in preceding sections that is key to such functional benefit.

• Reduction of unnecessary complications. The disabled person can easily run into unnecessary and additional problems as a result of unrecognized or untreated complications. Untreated spasticity, for example, can lead to muscle contracture which further worsens functionality, increases dependency, and places the person at a risk of even more complications, such as pressure sores. Other significant problems can arise, for example, with inappropriately treated incontinence or unrecognized depression. The following sections in the book will outline many such examples.

• Better coordination and use of resources. The person with complex and severe disabilities needs a variety of health, social, and other services. There is the clear potential for unnecessary overlap of assessment, treatment, and follow-up. The rehabilitation team should act as a single point of contact and a single point of information for the disabled person and their family. The team should be in the best position to coordinate the various services. Many people with complex disabilities now have the benefit of a case manager whose key role is to coordinate the different health and social inputs. Ideally the disabled person or a key family member should act in this role but this is not always possible, particularly for those people with residual cognitive or intellectual challenges.

• Cost-effective use of resources. Unfortunately there are few studies that confirm the cost benefits of rehabilitation. There are some studies which, in general, have shown such benefits. In Newcastle upon Tyne in the UK, for example, a multidisciplinary multiple sclerosis team was established in the city. The economic benefits, in terms of reduced hospital bed usage and reduced outpatient visits, were offset by the cost of the team itself so that the whole team was introduced as a cost-neutral venture. It seems self-evident, although research is still needed, that better functional gains and avoidance of unnecessary complications should make the best use of scarce health and social resources. If a disabled person can be assisted back to work, even on a part-time basis, then it is a major cost saving for the national economy. About 80% of the costs of disability are due to lost employment opportunities.

- Education, training, and research. There is a need for further studies in the whole realm of rehabilitation. Much more education, training, and research is needed. A rehabilitation team can act in such an education and research capacity and can help to enhance knowledge, reduce ignorance, and go some way to reducing the discrimination in disability.

Summary

This introductory section has outlined the concepts, principles, and processes of rehabilitation and illustrated some of the benefits. It is a process of education and enablement that centrally involves the disabled person and the family. It is a process that must be conducted through a series of specific goals on route to a long-term strategic aim. We now know that rehabilitation can produce real benefit in terms of functional improvement, fewer unnecessary complications, better coordination of services, and cost-effectiveness as well as providing a key role in general education, training, and research for both professionals and disabled people.

In summary the basic tasks of rehabilitation are:

- To work in partnership with the disabled person and their family.
- To give accurate information and advice about the nature of the disability, natural history, prognosis, etc.
- To listen to the needs and perceptions of the disabled person and the family.
- To assist in the establishment of realistic rehabilitation goals appropriate to that person's disability, family, social, and employment needs.
- To establish appropriate measures so that the disabled person and the rehabilitation team know when such goals have been obtained.
- To work with all colleagues in an interdisciplinary fashion.
- To liaise as needed with carers and advocates of the disabled person.
- To foster appropriate education and training of health and social service professionals as well as helping to meet the educational requirements of the disabled person.
- To foster research, both quantitative and qualitative, into the many aspects of the rehabilitation service—from scientific principles to the basic service delivery.

Rehabilitation has in the past been viewed as a rather vague and woolly process—often with justification. However, modern rehabilitation should be a combination of a precise science and the art of traditional medicine.

Recommended further reading

1 Barnes, M.P. and Ward, A.B. (2000) *Textbook of Rehabilitation Medicine*. Oxford University Press, Oxford.

2 Brisenden, S. (1986). Independent living in the medical model. *Disability, Handicap and Society* **1**, 173–8.

3 Dobkin, B.H. (ed.). (2003). *The Clinical Science of Neurologic Rehabilitation*, 2nd edn. Oxford University Press, Oxford.

4 Greenwood, R.J., Barnes, M.P., MacMillan, T.M., and Ward, C.D. (eds). (2003). *Handbook of Neurological Rehabilitation*. Psychology Press, Hove.

5 Wade, D.T. (ed.). (1996). *Measurement in Neurological Rehabilitation*. Oxford University Press, Oxford.

Epidemiology

Epidemiology is the study of patterns of the occurrence of disease in populations and of factors that influence these patterns. It may seem strange to discuss this early in the book, but such discussion puts the whole issue of disability into perspective, and also places individual conditions in perspective. Knowledge of epidemiology is linked to the natural history of a disease or condition, and is therefore relevant to clinical practice.

Incidence and prevalence of a condition

Incidence is the number of new cases appearing in a unit time, e.g. per year. *Prevalence* is the number of affected people in community at any one time (6 million disabled people in the UK).
- Differences between the two may be small or large depending on the survival of patients.
- Conditions with a high prevalence may have a significant impact on resource allocation, e.g. osteoarthritis, stroke, traumatic brain injury.
- Rapidly progressive problems, e.g. cancers and motor neuron disease, require rapid flexible responses in the knowledge that service provision may require change after only a short time.
- Rehabilitation services are more concerned with prevalence than with incidence.

Disability is common (Table 2.1), with 14% of the adult population of the UK having a disability. The prevalence of disability among adults aged 16 years and over was 135 per 1000 population and, if one includes those people living in institutions, the prevalence increases to 142 per 1000. Seventy-seven per cent of disabled people were found to have one or more of the physical disabilities, implying a prevalence rate of 104.1 per 1000 aged 16 years and over, living in the community, and 109 per 1000, including those living in institutions. Although locomotion disability is the most common for all age groups the combination of physical and mental disabilities appears to be the most disabling.

Table 2.1 Disability domains—estimates of prevalence of disability in Great Britain by type (ICIDH) and age per 1000 population

Type of disability	Age group 16–59	60–74	75+	All adults
Locomotion	31	198	496	99
Hearing	17	110	328	59
Personal care	18	99	313	57
Dexterity	13	78	199	40
Seeing	9	56	262	38
Intellectual function	20	40	109	34
Behaviour	19	40	152	31
Reaching and stretching	9	54	149	28
Communication	12	42	140	27
Continence	9	42	147	26
Disfigurement	5	18	27	9
Eating, drinking, and digesting	2	12	30	6
Consciousness	5	10	9	5

From Martin, J., Meltzer, H. and Elliot, D. (1988). *The Prevalence of Disability among Adults*, OPCS Report 1. HMSO, London.

International Classification of Functioning and Health (ICF)

The World Health Organization published the International Classification of Impairments, Disability, and Handicap (ICIDH) in 1980 as part of its preparation for the International Year for the Disabled in 1981. This was widely adopted in clinical practice and became established as a means to initiate the rehabilitation process. However, over the ensuing years its shortcomings became apparent, particularly when disabled people were clinically managed in different settings. In addition, it was seen as negative and highlighted a person's dependence. As a result, a further classification was produced in 1997, in which the disability and handicap domains were replaced by the more positive terms of 'activity' and 'participation'. This still did not go far enough in recognizing the impact of disability on a person's life and did not translate from health care to social aspects of life. The ICF was thus established in 2001 and attempts to add personal and environmental factors, which have an important role in the perception of limitations to functioning and participation (Fig. 2.1). It recognizes the impact of disease on a person's functioning in terms of loss of organ function and thus functioning, but also associates this with loss of personal functioning and limitation of participation. Just because a person has an impairment, e.g. a foot drop, it does not mean that he or she is limited in activities and in participation. It depends on the context of a person's life and on the surrounding environment. For instance, this impairment may only have a small impact on the participation of a middle-aged professional person working in an office, but would probably be profoundly limiting on a manual worker or a professional sportsman.

Human experience of disablement

Fig. 2.1 The ICF classification of disability.

Application of the Office for Population Censuses and Surveys (OPCS)

The OPCS conducted a major survey of disability in 1988 and 1989, which has given a fundamental view on the lives of disabled people living in the UK. Similar censuses have been conducted elsewhere, but the OPCS produced a tool whereby the impact of disability could be measured in terms of personal functioning and participation in daily life (Table 2.2).

In the UK most disability is due to musculoskeletal disease and is followed by problems related to the eye and ear (Table 2.3). Generally speaking, neurological conditions make up a smaller component, but have far greater relevance in the more severe categories of disability on the OPCS scale. In fact, severe disability in younger people is primarily due to neurological disease.

Severe disability is also associated with multiple pathology, and people over 60 years of age are more likely to have two or more conditions, which increase in severity with age. Arthritis and hypertension, the two conditions with the highest prevalence, coexisted in over one-quarter of those aged 60 years and over. Because of this association with co-morbid disease, there exists an essential difference between the rehabilitation of older people compared with younger groups. Certain conditions are more prevalent in different parts of the country—e.g. multiple sclerosis increases as one moves north throughout the UK—and services have to reflect the needs of local populations. In addition, the affluence and social circumstances of certain parts of the UK appears to be reflected by a concomitant change in the levels of disability and disadvantage, and this is perhaps based on occupational factors and different levels of educational attainment and income.

Table 2.2 OPCS classification by type and severity of disability

Type of disability	Severity (%) 1–2	3–4	5–6	7–8	9–10	Total
Other disability (not physical)	38	26	17	5	0	23
Physical	39	35	31	25	18	33
Physical and sensory	21	31	30	36	28	28
Physical and mental (±sensory)	2	8	24	34	56	18
Total	100	100	100	100	100	100

From Martin, J., White, A., and Meltzer, H. (1989). *Disabled Adults, Services, Transport and Employment*. OPCS Report 4. HMSO, London.

Table 2.3 Frequency of disease groups causing physical disabilities and all disability—adults in private households (per 1000 population)

Disease ICD group	Type of disability All types	Locomotor	Reaching and stretching	Dexterity	Disfigurement
Musculoskeletal	46	56	64	67	61
Ear	38	1	0	0	1
Eye	22	2	0	1	2
Circulatory	20	23	10	7	5
Mental	13	3	2	3	1
Nervous system	13	12	21	22	12
Respiratory	13	14	3	2	1
Digestive	6	2	2	1	5
Genitourinary	3	1	1	0	2
Neoplasms	2	1	3	2	4
Endocrine	2	2	1	1	1
Infections	1	1	1	1	3
Blood	1	0	0	0	0
Skin	1	1	0	0	4
Congenital	0	0	0	0	3
Other	6	5	3	4	1

From Martin, J., White, A., and Meltzer, H. (1989). *Disabled Adults, Services, Transport and Employment*. OPCS Report 4. HMSO, London.

How does epidemiological information help us?

It is important in rehabilitation medicine to know whether one is trying to change a person's impairment, functioning, or participation. For instance, if the goal of rehabilitation is to allow a person with impaired mobility to get upstairs to use the bathroom, one could approach the problem in three ways:

- Definitive treatment could be directed at the pathology and impairment to diminish their effects and restore function in the limbs.
- Functioning could be addressed with the result that, despite a continuing impairment, the person could be trained to climb the stairs and walk to the bathroom.
- A chair lift and a wheelchair could be provided, such that the person could be transported upstairs, transferred to a wheelchair at the top of the stairs, and then either be taken or take themselves to the bathroom.

Although the ultimate aim would be the same, the options would involve different activities by different people at different levels and with a different impact on the disabled person and their family.

Participation is quite the most difficult domain to address, as it varies from person to person, according to their circumstances, and is often outwith the control of the health-based rehabilitation team. A disabled person's life satisfaction is most difficult to measure, as reduced participation is not an inevitable and direct consequence of impairment and disability. It actually arises from an interaction of the impairment and functioning with other external factors, such as the home environment, the job, personal relations, etc. Its impact derives from society's general attitude to disabled people and it is influenced by culture and by society's values and expectations. For instance, the expectations of the parents of disabled adolescents are significantly lower where there is a congenital disability (or one from a very early age) rather than an acquired disability. The impact of a physical disability on the life of an individual is therefore not just related to the disease process or to the number of individual disabilities, but to what are termed as contextual factors. These include orientation, physical independence, mobility, occupation, social integration, and economic self-sufficiency and Badley's model (1995) encapsulates this (Fig. 2.2). Many people can be severely affected by disability but are quite satisfied with their lifestyles, whereas others, with similar or lesser disabilities, may be unable to exist.

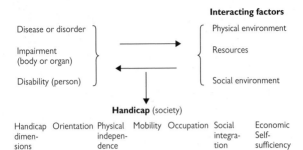

Fig. 2.2 A model for the consequences of disease, disorders, or injuries (after Badley and Tennant 1997).

The rehabilitation team

Rehabilitation teams

Rehabilitation is about team work. It is a process that has to involve a wide range of different professionals. Rehabilitation teams can work in many different contexts. Many teams will be hospital based and working primarily with people after a stroke or traumatic brain injury. Such teams will mainly involve physicians, therapists, and nurses. However, other teams can work in a different context and team membership will have a different emphasis. A community rehabilitation team is more likely to involve local authority employees, such as social workers and community occupational therapists, and perhaps other professionals, such as employment experts. Thus, it is not possible, or indeed desirable, to define disciplines that must be members of a rehabilitation team. Indeed a list of such disciplines will inappropriately emphasize professional boundaries. The essence of the rehabilitation team is that it is not simply a collection of different professionals but a coherent group of such professionals working together for the common good of the disabled person. A simple collection of appropriate professionals could be called a *multidisciplinary team*. Whilst such a team may contain the necessary range of professionals evidence shows that such a team does not produce the necessary benefits that should flow from the rehabilitation process. The rehabilitation team must function as a coherent whole so that client-centred goals can be set and monitored and such goals should cross traditional professional boundaries. The team should not be *discipline orientated* but *outcome orientated*.

There is extensive literature on the definition of teams but the following list (after Furnell et al.[1]) provides a useful summary of the main characteristics of a rehabilitation team:

- Professionals from different disciplines who meet regularly.
- The allocation, by each member, of a significant proportion of his/her own time to the pursuit of a team's objectives.
- Agreement on explicit objectives for the team that determine the team's structure and function.
- Adequate administrative and clinical coordination to support the work of the team, although not necessarily by the same person on all occasions.
- A defined geographical base.
- A clear differentiation of and respect for those skills and roles that are specific and unique to individual members as well as recognition of those roles that may be shared.

Why have teams?

There is evidence that a proper rehabilitation team can produce functional benefit for the disabled person over and above a collection of individuals working together as a group. Some of the benefits of such team work are likely to be:[2]

- Improved communication.
- Sharing of knowledge between people of different disciplines.
- A more consistent goal-orientated approach and better continuity of care.
- Promotion of a broad perspective for rehabilitation provision.
- Provision of a stimulating environment to enhance the contribution of team members, improve motivation, and increase individual effectiveness.
- Creation of an 'esprit de corps' that leads to a mutually supporting atmosphere.

These characteristics are useful as they emphasize not only the importance of the rehabilitation team for the disabled person but also the importance of the team for its constituent members. Rehabilitation is a broad subject and no individual can carry all the necessary knowledge and information required to provide a cohesive and thorough rehabilitation programme. Single practitioners working by themselves, often in the community, can begin to feel lonely and isolated and part of a team function is mutual support, recognition of problems, and development of a team culture where no one individual feels isolated or overwhelmed.

Interdisciplinary teams

The essence of rehabilitation is the focusing of goal setting and the needs of a particular individual with a disability. Individuals rarely package their particular requirements into neat professional boundaries. An individual will rarely say that he or she has a specific physiotherapy goal or an occupational therapy goal or a clinical psychology goal. The individual's goals are most likely to cross professional boundaries. A rehabilitation team must recognize the importance of such client-centred goals and adjust their own work patterns accordingly. If, for example, a long-term goal is to walk independently then an appropriate subgoal may be to negotiate a flight of stairs independently, in a particular fashion. The physiotherapist is likely to be the key team member that works with the disabled person in achieving this goal. However, it is still the responsibility of the other team members to heed the advice of the physiotherapist and work with the client to achieve that particular aim. The speech therapist, leading the person to a speech therapy session up a flight of stairs, will need to be aware of the stair-climbing technique just as much as the physiotherapist will need to be aware of the communication strategy that might be led by the speech therapist.

This approach is termed *interdisciplinary working*. The members of the rehabilitation team will need to flexible and prepared to work across artificial professional boundaries. 'That's not my job' is not an attitude required in a rehabilitation team. Interdisciplinary working implies a blurring of professional roles whilst still preserving the separate identity and expertise of individual professions. The ultimate goal of this approach is to produce an integrated assessment and to develop a unified treatment plan that is jointly carried out by all team members. Thus, it demands a higher degree of group interaction and focused treatment effort than a simple multidisciplinary team. It is also a team that should incorporate the disabled person and their family as part of the team itself. It is equally important for family members to understand the goals and the methods by which they are being achieved. Such understanding can only come if the family is an integral part of the rehabilitation team.

Generic rehabilitation workers

This is a concept in rehabilitation that is gathering momentum. The ultimate role extension must be to completely blur professional boundaries. Such therapists are no longer identified as physiotherapists, occupational therapists, or clinical psychologists but simply co-partners in a rehabilitation team. This ultimate approach implies a broad-based generic training which currently does not exist (except perhaps in the somewhat artificial environment of conductive education as practiced in the Peto Institute in Budapest and other centres). This is probably a model that works better in the context of the rehabilitation of neurobehavioural problems after traumatic brain injury. This type of rehabilitation, especially in the later stages of recovery, requires a particular emphasis on communication and coordination of care so that the individual has a coordinated, well-documented, and consistent response to various behavioural problems. The members of such a team, often led by a clinical neuropsychologist, work in a *transdisciplinary* fashion where professional boundaries are no longer recognized. However, the neurobehavioural team is a specific example and it may be very difficult, and perhaps inappropriate, to apply this in a more traditional post-acute rehabilitation unit. Nevertheless, in such units most of the day-to-day rehabilitation can be carried out by *generic health-care workers* who work under the guidance of the qualified therapist. These generic assistants often take on the role of a keyworker and are the main point of contact between the disabled person and a broader-based team. There are many different models. In some centres such an assistant takes on an important coordinating and educational role for the disabled person whilst in other centres the assistant is more subsidiary to the qualified therapist. Regrettably there is little research that enables meaningful comparisons to be made between different models of rehabilitation team working.

Keyworker or case manager

Whatever model of working is adopted by the rehabilitation team there are always a large number of individuals who need to liaise with the disabled person. This can produce a sense of confusion or a lack of direction. Teams have developed different ways around this problem. A common system is the allocation of a *keyworker*. One team member is allocated to be the key liaison between the team, the disabled person, and the family. The keyworker acts as the main source of information about the rehabilitation process and feeds back the thoughts and aspirations of the disabled person to the team, and vice versa. This system should not be seen as a substitute for regular team meetings nor should there be an abrogation of responsibility by relevant professionals. It is simply part of the whole rehabilitation team process that may lead to better coordination and liaison and clear channels of communication. In theory the keyworker can be any team member as long as that individual has an appropriate range of interpersonal skills and broad background knowledge of the needs and requirements of the disabled person. In many cases it would be entirely appropriate for the disabled person him/herself to act as the keyworker. However, this is not always possible, particularly if the person has troublesome cognitive and intellectual problems. If an advocate is required it is probably inappropriate for the advocate to act as the keyworker. The role of the advocate is purely to advocate the cause of the disabled person whereas the role of a keyworker is often one of negotiation and arbitration when opinions and goals diverge or are felt to be unrealistic.

In some cases the role of the keyworker can be extended to that of a *case manager*. The concept of case management has been developed as a way of assisting disabled people with the coordination of the necessary professional staff. Case management can include:

- Simple coordination within a single agency.
- Coordination across agency boundaries.
- Service brokerage in which the case manager negotiates with the key agencies on the client's behalf.
- Budget holding responsibility where services can be purchased on behalf of the client from statutory bodies or other voluntary and private agencies.

Although there have been few controlled studies of the efficacy of case management it is now a widely practised role and almost certainly provides a better and more coherent service and assists people, particularly those with cognitive impairment, to find their way through the maze of services. Indeed the role of case manager is now being seen as a separate and valid profession and care must be taken to ensure that a professional role designed to reduce and cross professional boundaries does not in itself produce a new professional discipline!

Core team

Despite the importance of interdisciplinary working there is still a core membership for a health-orientated rehabilitation team. Core members of the team are:

- rehabilitation nurse
- clinical neuropsychologist
- occupational therapist
- physiotherapist
- speech and language therapist
- rehabilitation physician.

It is difficult to envisage a post-acute rehabilitation team that does not have access to such individuals. However, the team will often need to draw on a wide range of other expertise, such as social work and counselling, as well as having occasional access to dieticians, chiropodists, and rehabilitation engineers. Sometimes access to other medical specialties is required, such as urology and orthopaedic surgery. In the community there often needs to be a broader network of core individuals. Health requirements quickly change to social requirements and input from social service occupational therapists and social workers soon becomes crucial. At later stages useful links can be fostered with employment rehabilitation experts as well as other voluntary providers, lawyers, social security staff, and a variety of disability support groups.

Thus, there is the concept of a *nuclear team* and the *support team*. The former comprises those people most involved with the individual on a day-to-day basis. The support team are more peripherally involved. The support team are usually not so 'hands on' and may not be in daily contact with either the disabled individual or the team. They could be said to act as consultants to the team rather than being intrinsic team members.

Team leadership

This can be a problem. The leader of many rehabilitation teams is the physician. This is usually for historical or political reasons and not necessarily because the doctor makes the best leader. Indeed it can be argued that medical training by its very nature encourages autonomous independent thinking in order to make quick decisions in acute situations and that this style is not best suited to the qualities required of a team leader. However, it has to be recognized that in many organizations, and in many cultures, it is not practical to suggest that anyone other than the doctor should lead the team. There are some advantages that medicine has over other specialisms. Medical training is able to give a broad overview of a particular disorder rather than the potentially narrower perspective of other professional disciplines. The doctor should be able to have a view of the 'whole person' with some grasp of the role of other professionals, and an understanding of the complementary role of team members can be a useful characteristic. However, the team leader needs to have other qualities. A leader has usefully been described as someone tolerant enough to listen to others but strong enough to reject their advice. The other characteristics that need to be displayed by a leader include:

- Good interpersonal and social skills.
- Vision for the long-term future of the team.
- Communication skills.
- Listening skills.
- Flexibility—the ability to listen to others and adjust the direction of the team according to the thoughts and views of other team members.
- Toughness—to make difficult decisions as and when they arise.
- Organizational skills.
- Good time management—to devote enough time to the team activities rather than just clinical tasks.
- Financial and budgetary understanding.
- Political skills—to influence colleagues and managers and direct maximum resources to the team.

It is doubtful whether such an individual exists who can fulfil all these criteria!

Whilst hospital-based teams are still usually under the direction of the hospital consultant there are now an increasing number of teams with non-medical team leaders, particularly in a community setting, or teams with an emphasis on the neurobehavioural and cognitive problems of disabled people.

Overall there is no doubt that the right leader is more important than their professional background.

References

1 Furnell, J., Flett, S., and Clarke, D.F. (1987). Multidisciplinary clinical teams: some issues in establishment and function. *Hospital and Health Services Review*, January, 15–18.

2 Wood, R.L. (2003). The rehabilitation team. In: *Handbook of Neurological Rehabilitation*, 2nd edn (ed. Greenwood, R.J., Barnes, M.P., McMillan, T.M., and Ward, C.D.), pp. 41–50. Psychology Press, Hove.

Chapter 4

Organization of services

Principles of service delivery

This section will look at the various organizational aspects of the delivery of a comprehensive rehabilitation service. There is no single way to develop a rehabilitation service and the physical base, team, structure, and scope and range of the services provided will clearly vary from community to community. This chapter will outline some of the possibilities for the organization of services and discuss the merits and drawbacks of different systems.

However, no matter how the team is structured it should first establish the basic principles under which it chooses to work. A useful set of principles was produced by the Prince of Wales Advisory Group on Disability in 1985. These are as follows:

- Disabled people and their family should be consulted as services are planned.
- Information should be clearly presented and readily available to all disabled consumers.
- The life of disabled people in the local and national community should be promoted with respect to both responsibilities and benefits.
- Disabled people should have a choice as to where to live and how to maintain independence, including help in learning how to choose.
- There should be recognition that long-term disability is not synonymous with illness and that the medical model of care is inappropriate in the majority of cases.
- The service should provide autonomy for the freedom to make decisions regarding a way of life best suited to an individual disabled person's circumstances.

Although not part of the Prince of Wales principles a seventh principle could be added:

- A fully comprehensive range of rehabilitation services should be provided as close to an individual's home as possible.

Most comprehensive rehabilitation systems are based on a two-tier service. Most rehabilitation can and should be carried out either at home or in the individual's own neighbourhood. Thus, each community should have an accessible and local rehabilitation team. However, it also has to be recognized that some disabled people, probably around 10%, will require the expertise and facilities of a more specialist service. Hopefully some elements of a specialist service can be delivered locally but almost certainly there will need to be a regional specialist rehabilitation centre to complement and supplement the services provided by the local team. The range and type of services required at a regional level and at a local level will obviously depend on the availability of appropriately trained staff, resources, and facilities and will vary from area to area. Close links between the regional services and the local services are vital. The disabled client should be able to move seamlessly from one service to the other with continuity of care, and preferably a local therapist should remain in touch with the client whilst the individual is within the regional centre and vice versa. However, resources are scarce and an ideal fully interlinked two-tier rehabilitation system is difficult to achieve.

Regional rehabilitation services

The regional specialist rehabilitation centre should work on the same underlying philosophy as any local team. It should work on the same principles of rehabilitation, particularly interdisciplinary team work, goal setting, and properly documented outcome measures. The regional team will consist of more specialist therapists, physicians, and nurses and will probably contain a more specialist range of equipment and assessment facilities. The population served by each centre will vary considerably according to the range and scope of the local team, of the local geography, and of the local resources. However, the following list of services should be provided from a regional centre as the skills or equipment required are unlikely to be available locally:

- A specialist rehabilitation service for people with the most complex multiple disabilities, particularly those with traumatic brain injury who have a combination of physical, psychological, and behavioural problems.
- A spinal injury service—in the UK there is a network of separate spinal injury regional centres, which developed historically under the original guidance of Sir Ludwig Guttman of Stoke Mandeville Hospital.
- A specialist service for complex wheelchair and special seating needs.
- A regional bioengineering service.
- A communication aids centre to provide specialist equipment for those with the most complicated communication problems.
- A centre for advice and assessment on assistive technology, particularly environmental control systems.
- An information, advice, and assessment service for car driving for disabled people.
- A service for amputees and adults and children with limb deformities (such as brachial plexus injuries, traumatic amputation, etc).
- An inpatient service for assessment and perhaps long-term care of people in prolonged coma, prolonged vegetative state, or a minimally conscious state.
- A range of specialist outpatient services that are not provided more locally. The range of outpatient support will vary considerably but potential services are likely to include the following:
  - Spasticity clinic.
  - Botulinum toxin injection service for spasticity and other conditions such as dystonia.
  - A sexual counselling and advice service for disabled people.
  - A specialist orthotic service.
  - Specialist neuropsychological clinics, particularly for those with cognitive, intellectual, and memory problems.
  - A specialist neurobehavioural service (both inpatient and outpatient), particularly for people with behavioural problems in the context of traumatic brain injury.

The regional centre should also be a focus for education and training for health professionals, both within the centre and for the local teams, and indeed other health and social services professionals around the region. Thus, lecture facilities and appropriate libraries and other internet resources should be provided.

Finally the regional centre could also act as a focus for rehabilitation research and a link with a local academic centre would be important.

The design of the regional centre is also important. It should include realistic assessment areas such as kitchens, bathrooms, toilets, and bedrooms. It should certainly have a wide range of specialist equipment, such as specialist wheelchairs and assistive technology for assessment and demonstration purposes. Outdoor areas need to be provided for outdoor walking training, with different surfaces, and probably a car driving track would be necessary for the range of driving adaptation equipment to be properly demonstrated. If disabled people and their families are travelling a considerable distance then suitable overnight facilities or facilities for relatives to stay for a period of time would also be desirable.

Local rehabilitation services

The local rehabilitation team should be able to deliver all standard post-acute inpatient rehabilitation for individuals in the locality. This would, for example, include a stroke unit. Most district general hospitals in the UK who take acute admissions now have some form of rehabilitation unit and indeed it is a requirement of the UK government that by 2004 all such hospitals must have a stroke rehabilitation unit. However, it is important that inpatient services for those with other post-acute rehabilitation requirements are not missed out, particularly for those people with more complex neurological problems such as moderate brain injury, multiple sclerosis, motor neuron disease, etc. An inpatient rehabilitation unit at a local level should clearly have close links, both clinical and educational, with a regional centre. A regional centre should be able to receive referrals from the local unit and once a particular problem has been successfully managed the individual should be sent back to the local inpatient unit and from there back into the community.

However, a local inpatient unit, whilst important, goes only a small way to meet all the health needs of disabled people in a locality. Most people after discharge from an inpatient unit will continue to have rehabilitation requirements. There are many disabled people who will never have an acute event (such as those with cerebral palsy, multiple sclerosis, etc) and thus would never come into contact with a hospital-based post-acute rehabilitation unit. There is an obvious need for a community focused, and preferably community-based, rehabilitation team. The various models of such services are described later in this section.

In specific terms a local rehabilitation team should be able to provide all or most of the following:

- An inpatient post-acute rehabilitation service—particularly after stroke and moderate traumatic brain injury as well as occasional assessment and respite facilities for those with progressive conditions such as multiple sclerosis.
- A service for people with continence problems.
- A local orthotic service.
- A local prescription and maintenance service for basic wheelchairs.
- A nursing-based service for those with pressure sores.
- A counselling service that helps individuals with adjustment and coping problems in the context of physical disability—including sexual counselling.
- An appropriate range of outpatient support services.
- A rehabilitation liaison service with the acute medical, surgical, and psychiatric wards for those with physical disabilities who require other hospital admission.
- An aids and equipment service, probably including local provision of environmental control equipment.
- A basic information and advice service.

The local team will need to maintain a broad network of contacts with other relevant professionals and departments, including the local authority social service department, housing department, local employment rehabilitation service, and social security office. Local disability groups should also be associated with the local team and can provide invaluable peer support and information.

Rehabilitation unit

The rehabilitation team will need a physical base. There are many advantages to the creation of a dedicated rehabilitation unit. A physical unit is obviously required for a post-acute inpatient facility. However, even a community-based team will need a physical base to provide rooms for seeing clients, displaying equipment, and putting on seminars as well as providing necessary administrative support. Thus, every locality should have a clearly identified physical base. Ideally the rehabilitation unit needs to have the following facilities:

- An appropriate number of inpatient beds—the figure will vary considerably according to local needs and resources but around 20 beds would probably meet the post-acute rehabilitation needs of the 16–65-year-old population with (post-acute) neurological disabilities for a population of around 250 000 people.
- Communal living spaces.
- Practice kitchen, bedroom, and living areas.
- A self-contained flat to allow further practice at daily living skills for individuals about to return to the community.
- Space for appropriate outpatient clinics—although many services ought to be provided either in the home or even more local facilities, such as the GP surgery or other community centre.
- Space for information displays.
- Seminar and teaching space as well as meeting areas for the local team and perhaps local voluntary and disability groups.
- Plenty of appropriate car parking and ready access to accessible transport links.

The unit itself should obviously be fully accessible for people with a whole range of disabilities.

The presence of a physical unit is likely to be conducive to the development of an identifiable rehabilitation team, which should promote staff morale and stimulate education, training, and research. There are advantages if the unit is based separately from acute hospital wards. Moving to a separate rehabilitation unit can be seen as a step towards return to the community and might allow for more appropriate 'non-hospital' design.

Organizational models—the outpatient clinic

Equal delivery of health care to the disabled population is a major logistical task. As 14% of the adult population have a disability and at least 2–3% of the population have a severe disability then it is clear that a local rehabilitation service will need to see a large number of people—many of whom will need to be seen on an on-going basis. There are many different models of service delivery and no single model is preferable to another. The service design must meet the local needs and take into account other local and regional resources, staffing, and facilities. Even in one area it is likely that several of the service models described in the next sections could apply.

The traditional model for short- and long-term support of people with disabilities is through the hospital outpatient clinic. The advantages of the outpatient service are:

- It is easier logistically to see people in one physical setting from the point of view of maximum use of staff time.
- It may be possible for the same inpatient team who looked after an individual in the post-acute setting to continue to see that individual on an outpatient basis—thus ensuring continuity of care.
- It may be possible to arrange outpatients so that individuals with the same sort of problem can attend for a particular clinic—for example, to provide a specific multiple sclerosis clinic or a Parkinson's disease clinic or alternatively symptom-based clinics such as an incontinence clinic or a spasticity clinic. This service would enable an expert multidisciplinary team to be on hand at each clinic and provide the necessary assessment and treatment as well as providing appropriate information and advice. Such a clinic could act as a focus for the relevant local self-help group.

However, there are a number of significant disadvantages to an outpatient system:

- The outpatient clinics often run on a medical model with junior medical staff seeing the individual—often for the first time and with little prior knowledge of the disability or circumstances.
- There is little time to spend with each individual.
- Reappointment intervals tend to be several months apart when shorter intervals are sometimes more appropriate.
- It may be difficult to involve other relevant members of the multidisciplinary team.
- Disease-specific clinics may provide logistical problems in arranging a sufficient number of such clinics to cover the necessary range of disabilities and symptoms and thus there is a risk of ignoring the needs of people with rarer conditions.
- Some find it distressing to see individuals with the same condition in a more disabled state.
- Outpatient clinics are generally regarded as unsatisfactory by the users and many disability publications confirm this point.

Organizational models—primary care team

A typical group general practice in the UK has a population of around 10 000 people. The numbers of people requiring assistance from a rehabilitation team are reduced to a manageable number if the team is based within a typical general practice population. The advantages of the rehabilitation team being general practice-based are:

- The rest of the primary care team are on hand to deal with other general medical problems as and when they arise.
- People with disabilities tend not to be seen as a separate specific entity but are seen as part of the general population simply attending the GP's surgery as any other member of the public.
- The GP's surgery would tend to be local and usually reasonably accessible for the disabled person.
- The knowledge of the local primary care team should be increased by contact with local rehabilitation professionals.

However, there are some clear disadvantages:

- Many disabilities are quite rare. The GP, for example, is likely to only see one new person with multiple sclerosis every 20 years. Thus the level of expertise within the primary care team is strictly limited and undoubtedly the primary care team would need to be supplemented with appropriately trained rehabilitation staff.
- It is unlikely that necessary expertise and rehabilitation professionals could be provided for every primary care team. Recruitment and retention could be major problems.
- The local rehabilitation team could feel professionally isolated and slowly become deskilled if inadequate attention is paid to appropriate links with local and regional teams as well as specific time put aside for education and training.

However, there are many ways where a primary care team can be involved in the long-term management of people with physical disabilities. In one project, for example, a rehabilitation physician and a physiotherapist attend regular meetings with the primary care team to discuss management issues for people with Parkinson's disease. In another project the specialist rehabilitation team does outreach clinics in a GP's surgery. In a further project, in a large group general practice, one GP and one district nurse have been specifically trained by the regional rehabilitation team to manage the more routine and day-to-day difficulties encountered by disabled people—thus providing some local specialist knowledge to the local disabled population.

Organizational models—community rehabilitation team

In theory a full interdisciplinary rehabilitation team could be provided in the local community. The team would clearly need close liaison and good working relations with the local primary care team in that area as well as the local hospital unit and indeed the regional unit. Such an arrangement should overcome some of the disadvantages of the service being provided by the primary care team itself. One example, in Newcastle upon Tyne, is a local community multiple sclerosis team. The team has a physical base in a local disabled living centre but assessment and on-going therapy is conducted in the individual's home. There is a weekly group physiotherapy session in a local day unit. The team itself, consisting of a physiotherapist (team manager), occupational therapist, therapy assistant, and secretary, are all employed on a full-time basis as well as part-time input from a counsellor, social worker, multiple sclerosis nurse, clinical neuropsychologist, and rehabilitation physician. The team has access to wider specialist support and respite beds are provided in a local rehabilitation centre. The team accepts referrals from a variety of sources, particularly GPs and neurologists as well as the local multiple sclerosis society (which part funds the team). The team has good links with local social services department and the necessity for double assessment by the health team and then the social services team is avoided. The potential disadvantages of such a team are:

- The team may have a health focus and thus less emphasis on important social and vocational issues.
- The team may only deal with a particular disability (such as multiple sclerosis) to the detriment of people with other diagnostic conditions.
- The provision of a comprehensive community rehabilitation team in every locality is unrealistic as sufficient numbers of trained staff would simply not be available—nor would there be the resources to pay for their services.

Organizational models—specialist therapists and nurses

If a full community rehabilitation team is unlikely to be provided in every locality then a somewhat less expensive possibility is to provide specially trained individual practitioners. In recent years there has been a growth of the concept of the specialist practitioner, particularly in a nursing context. There are now specially trained nurses with expertise in such conditions as Parkinson's disease, epilepsy, and multiple sclerosis as well as symptom-based specialist nurses working in the fields of, for example, continence and stoma care. There is now the emerging concept of a similar specialist therapist—such as physiotherapists with a particular expertise in the management of spasticity. While some of these specialist therapists and nurses are still hospital based many are now beginning to work in a community setting. Some are attached to the primary care team whilst others perform outreach work from the local, or the regional, rehabilitation centres. There are a number of advantages to this model:

- A broad range of disorders and symptoms could be covered.
- It is clearly less expensive to provide a single broadly trained practitioner in the community rather than the full community rehabilitation team.
- The practitioner can act as a contact point for people within their expert area. Many problems should be able to be dealt with by the practitioner, but onward referral to the local or regional teams could still be made.
- Close links could be maintained with the primary care team.
- Disabled people could be seen in their own home—thus saving unnecessary trips to hospital outpatient departments or unnecessary hospital admission.

However, there are obvious disadvantages:

- One individual cannot provide all the necessary expertise to an entire diagnostic group.
- Individuals are working in isolation and do not have the advantages of working as a member of an interdisciplinary rehabilitation team.
- Individuals would require lengthy training and considerable effort would need to expended on continuing professional development. At the moment, at least in the UK, such comprehensive training and support programmes are not yet widely available.

Given relatively limited resources in health, however, the concept of the independent specialist practitioner working in the community that links to the local and regional centre is a model worth pursuing as long as such development goes hand in hand with a proper high-quality training programme.

Organizational models—the Independent Living Movement and resource centres

There are now many examples of local authorities giving disabled people their own budget to buy in their own services. This is a model firmly supported by the *Independent Living Movement* and by disabled groups in general. A disabled individual will access their own appropriate parts of the community rehabilitation team and buy in their care within their own home. This is certainly a workable solution for many disabled people. However, problems do arise in some circumstances. People with cognitive or behavioural problems may have difficulty identifying their own requirements. This can raise difficult questions—who should manage their affairs and who should judge whether a given individual is able to manage their own budget or not? If an advocate is needed then such an advocate will need appropriate training so they know which services are on offer and which are appropriate. How does the system deal with inappropriate or unprovidable purchasing requests? What happens if there insufficient funds or an individual's budget becomes overspent? There are solutions to all these questions, and indeed this model can work quite well for many people. However, for everyone to buy in all the services they require will clearly need a very significant increase in available resources for the disabled population and difficulties with rationing would soon come into play.

If some facilities could be shared then this may alleviate some problems. One solution is to provide a *local community resource centre*. Such centres would be local, accessible, and house a range of facilities, including an information service and a disabled living centre, and would probably act as a base for local voluntary and self-help groups as well as a physical site for the local rehabilitation team. Outpatient clinics could be held in the centre from the local hospital or indeed outreach clinics from the regional centre. Social and recreational activities could be provided and other agencies could have an office in the centre, such as housing, social security, and employment services. The centres could, and probably should, be managed by and for disabled people. A number of such resource centres have now been established in the UK and abroad.

Community rehabilitation in developing countries

Most of the examples in the preceding sections are applicable to health systems in the Western world, particularly in Europe, the USA, Australia, and Canada. However, most of the rest of the world has less than adequate rehabilitation resources and facilities. Many people in developing countries have no access at all to any rehabilitation facility. If they are able to get in to a hospital rehabilitation unit then more often than not there is no community support after discharge. Thus, other models have been developed to overcome these difficulties in the developing world. The World Health Organization developed the concept of *community based rehabilitation* (CBR). The model is open to different interpretations but the general approach is for the local community to be the main supporter of its own disabled population. Local village workers are given some basic disability training—perhaps just lasting a few weeks. In many parts of the world one or more individuals in the local village are already involved in some aspect of basic health care or child birth. These people are given further training, generally supported by non-governmental organizations, and are provided with further background disability knowledge. At this basic level of training it has been shown that such people can deal with about 80% of the needs of a disabled population in their own village. The village workers may need support and on-going training and supervision which is usually provided by a more trained individual who covers a number of local villages—perhaps visiting them on a regular basis to deal with more complex problems and make appropriate referrals to the local hospital or a regional centre.

The CBR model has been developed in many places to establish disabled groups in individual villages to provide economically viable employment for themselves. The groups, perhaps with some external support, are trained and provided with basic tools for such skills as woodworking, dressmaking, and bicycle repairing. These groups then contribute a small sum to a central pool so that a few members of the group needing medicine or external referral can be supported. Obviously such basic training and support of disabled people is far from ideal but nevertheless such systems have been shown to be viable, cheap, and offer sustainable solutions for many disabled people in terms of health care and employment. The concept also goes some way to reducing the stigma of disablity; disabled people in many cultures are marginalized from their own communities. There is a great need for much more to be done on a global basis and very significant investment is required in developing countries for the establishment of an appropriate disability infrastructure. However, CBR is a start and in many parts of the world is still the only means of long term support for disabled people.

Chapter 5

Assessment of disability

Why is disability assessment necessary?

Rehabilitation is a very complex activity and is difficult to quantify. Outcome measurement lacks the specificity seen in the treatment of pathology, but new thinking has brought new ways of assessing the issue. Rather than measure the activity of a pathology or disease, the focus is on the change due to the rehabilitation process, i.e. the added value of the rehabilitation given to a patient over and above a spontaneous recovery or improvement following an acute single injury or illness. Rehabilitation may slow down the deterioration and improve quality of life in patients with progressive disability, for which the measures used for static or improving conditions will not be appropriate. There are essentially five categories of patients:

1. Patients with potential to make a spontaneous full return to pre-morbid levels of health.
2. Steadily improving patients, but who may not return to pre-morbid levels of health and function.
3. Patients not improving greatly, but with potential to improve.
4. Slowly deteriorating patients, whose deterioration will be slowed by treatment and rehabilitation.
5. Steadily or rapidly deteriorating patients, despite rehabilitation interventions.

Rehabilitation is effective in all, but rehabilitation units have to design different programmes for each group. Measurement is thus important at a patient level to note a change in functioning, as well as at a health policy service level to assist in allocating funding for services. The International Classification of Functioning and Health allows rehabilitation issues to be assessed for changes in impairments and functioning within the contextual factors for any patient or population of people at risk.

Measurement

The following terms can be defined:
- *Measurement*: the use of a standard to quantify an observation.
- *Measurement tools*: the techniques used to quantify that observation.
- *Outcome*: the result obtained in using such instruments.

The essential measure in rehabilitation is to define the goals of rehabilitation for a particular patient and to determine whether or not the patient achieved the goal at the end of the rehabilitation episode. This is a measure of success, but the true value depends on the skill of the team in defining realistic, achievable, and desirable targets. If a goal is too easy, then the measure will have a ceiling effect, i.e. too many people will achieve the goal or the top of the scale, whereas if it is too difficult, the patient's actual achievements will not be amply recognized. Linear quantitative measures are *nominal*, *ordinal*, *interval*, *ratio* and *hierarchical*:

- Nominal scale: classifies a characteristic number along a straight line. Points on the scale have no meaning within the context in which they are being used, but may be useful if the frequencies of that particular characteristic are being studied.
- Ordinal scale: ranks the order, so that each adjacent score measures a parameter along a line, i.e. one point above or below is higher or lower than the last. Examples of this type of scale are the Visual Analogue Scale and the Barthel Index and Functional Independence Measurements.
- Interval scale: intervals sales have a common interval—i.e. a constant unit of measurement between one point and another—with an arbitrary zero point (as perhaps are the units of measurement).
- Ratio scale: an interval scale with a true zero at its origin, e.g. measuring weight or cost per case.
- Hierarchical scale: a natural hierarchy, e.g. each point on a rising scale indicates a greater ability or skill than the last.

The ideal scale should be sensitive, specific, reliable, appropriate, acceptable, and robust. Each must be validated against standard criteria to which the attribute may be assessed. In disability research, false positive and false negative findings are common, and a true positive rate (the sensitivity) needs to be compared against the false positive rate (i.e. the specificity). Not only must scores be valid, they must be reliable and consistent. They must also be reliable between raters as well as repeatable, so inter-rater reliability and test–retest reliability are of importance.

Examples

Examples of the scales used to measure different disability domains are given in Table 5.1. Tables 5.2 and 5.3 detail the MRC Scale and the Modified Ashworth Scale respectively.

Communication

Dysphasia can be screened using the Frenchay Aphasia Screening Test (FAST). This measures the ability to record a set of pictures and is a clinically useful bedside test. It correlates with the Boston Aphasia Screening Test, which is regularly used by speech and language therapists.

Cognitive measures

The Mini-Mental State Examination is widely used as screening test of cognitive impairment. It includes an assessment of many elements of higher cerebral functions, such as memory, attention, and language. It is a useful basic tool for inclusion in a battery of tests of cognitive function. However, the Hodkinson Mental Test and the digit span which is a test of attention within the Weschler Adult Intelligence Scale (WAIS) are valuable at the bedside.

In the Hodkinson Mental Test the patient scores 1 for correct answers to the following questions:
- Patient's age
- Time (to nearest hour)
- An address given for recall at the end of the test
- Name of hospital/area of town
- Year
- Month
- Patient's date of birth
- Date of a significant event, e.g. World War II
- Name of monarch/Prime Minister
- Count backwards from 20 to 1 (no errors but may correct self).

The Hospital Anxiety and Depression Scale is useful in stroke rehabilitation, but its value diminishes thereafter. A score of 7 or below for anxiety/depression is normal, though scores of 11 or above are abnormal.

Activities of Daily Living (ADL)—Modified Barthel Index

This has been validated in stroke: it is predictive at 1 month for functional independence at 6 months. It does not take into account difficulties with communication, cognition, and mood, but is simple, reliable, and quick to carry out. It should measure what the patient does do rather than what he or she can do, and thus an element of hierarchical significance appears. Total score can be up to 20 (see Tables 5.4 and 5.5).

The Functional Independence Measure (FIM) has 18 subsets measured on a scale of 1 to 7 (1 being total care required to 7 being full independence). The Functional Assessment Measure (FAM) has been added to the FIM to accommodate the burden of care in traumatic brain injury. This uses the same criteria but the FAM measures extend activities of daily living to cover community mobility and cognitive features which are relevant to post-acute traumatic brain injury rehabilitation. The FIM + FAM is only validated for inpatient settings and is designed to be performed by the whole rehabilitation team. It is also designed to give information for the planning of rehabilitation goals, and scores can be displayed in such a way that deficits can be easily identified. Rehabilitation units in the UK are gaining experience with this measure and it has become one of a basket of measures undertaken.

Participation

Several scales have been derived from the original WHO ICIDH text referring to orientation, physical independence, mobility, occupation, social integration, and economic self-sufficiency, of which the London Handicap Scale and the Edinburgh Rehabilitation Status Scale have become the best known. The Frenchay Activities Index measures social integration (a measure of a person's behaviour and therefore, in the absence of mental illness or a personality disorder, a useful measure of social function) also describes this aspect of life. Well-being is difficult to measure in either health or social settings and many profiles have been devised to identify subjective views on how well people feel and how satisfied they are with life. The Sickness Impact Profile and the SF36 are two which have been recommended, and the latter has been used widely in patients with musculoskeletal problems.

Table 5.1 Scales used to measure different disability domains

Domain	Impairment	Function and participation
Mobility	Power, e.g. MRC Scale. Spasticity (Ashworth and Tardieu Scales, Wartenburg Test, Motricity Index (lower and upper limb))	Walking speed and distance/time, 'time to get up and go' test
Upper limb and hand	Grip strength: dynamometry is crude, but simple to perform; using a small cuff and sphygmomanometer is useful in clinical practice	Nine hole peg test: assesses the ability to perform coordinated fine movements. It measures the time taken to place nine pegs in nine holes. The test should be terminated if it is not completed in 50s
Function	Physiological cost index (PCI) = (activity pulse rate−rest rate)/speed of activity	
Communication	Frenchay Aphasia Screening Test (FAST), Boston Aphasia Screening Test	
Cognition	Mini-Mental State Examination, Hodkinson Mental Test Score	Digit span: a test of attention within the Weschler Adult Intelligence Scale (WAIS)
Mood	Hospital Anxiety and Depression Test	
Disability	Activities of daily living	OPCS Disability Scale, Barthel Score, Functional Independence Measure (FIM), Nottingham Extended ADL Scale, London Handicap Scale, Sickness Impact Scale

Table 5.2 The MRC Scale

0	No muscular activity
1	Minimal contraction of muscle but insufficient to move a joint
2	Contraction of muscle sufficient to move a joint but not oppose gravity
3	Muscle contraction sufficient to move a joint against gravity, but not against physical resistance
4	Muscle contraction sufficient to move a joint against gravity and against mild/moderate resistance
5	Normal power, i.e. muscular contraction sufficient to resist firm resistance

Table 5.3 The Modified Ashworth Scale

4	Rigid extremity
3	Loss of full joint movement, difficult movement, considerable tone
2	Full joint/limb movement, but more marked increase in tone, limb still easily moved
1+	Slight increase in tone, catch and resistance throughout range of movement
1	Slight increase in tone, catch, or minimal resistance at end of range of movement
0	No increase in tone

Adapted from Bohannon, R.W. and Smith, M.B. (1986). *Physical Therapy* **67**, 206–7.

Table 5.4 Modified Barthel Index

Task	Score	Description
Bowels	0	Incontinent (or needs enemas)
	1	Occasional accident (once a week)
	2	Continent
Bladder	0	Incontinent/catheterized
	1	Occasional accident (max. once/24 h)
	2	Continent
Grooming	0	Needs help with personal care
	1	Independent face/hair/teeth/shaving
Toilet use	0	Dependent
	1	Needs help but can do something alone
	2	Independent (on and off, dressing, wiping)
Feeding	0	Unable
	1	Needs help with cutting, spreading etc.
	2	Independent
Transfer	0	Unable, no sitting balance
	1	Major help from 1 or 2 people, can sit
	2	Minor help (verbal or physical)
	3	Independent
Mobility	0	Immobile
	1	Wheelchair independent, including corners
	2	Walks with help of 1 person (verbal/physical)
	3	Independent but may use any aid
Stairs	0	Unable
	1	Needs help (verbal, physical)
	2	Independent
Dressing	0	Dependent
	1	Needs help but can do half unaided
	2	Independent including buttons, zips, laces etc.
Bathing	0	Dependent
	1	Independent or in shower

Table 5.5 Nottingham Extended ADL Index

Activity	Questions (Do you...?)	Not at all	With help	Alone with difficulty	Alone easily
Mobility	Walk around outside? Climb stairs? Get in and out of the car? Walk over uneven ground? Cross roads? Travel on public transport?				
Kitchen	Manage to feed yourself? Manage to make yourself a hot drink? Take hot drinks from one room to another? Do the washing up? Make yourself a hot snack?				
Domestic tasks	Manage your own money when you are out? Wash small items of clothing? Do a full clothes wash?				
Leisure activity	Read newspapers or books? Use the telephone? Write letters? Go out socially? Manager your own garden? Drive a car?				

Scoring: 0 = not at all/with help; 1 = alone with difficulty/alone easily.

Suggested further reading

1 Wade, D.T. (1992). *Measurement in Neurological Rehabilitation*. Oxford University Press, Oxford.

Spasticity

Definition

Spasticity is one of the most commonly encountered problems in the field of neurological rehabilitation. It is a significant factor that can reduce functional mobility and is a major impediment in the rehabilitation process. Untreated or badly treated spasticity can lead to joint contractures which in turn cause problems in maintaining a suitable posture for feeding, communication, and many aspects of daily living. Muscle spasms, often associated with spasticity, can be painful and one of the predisposing causes for the development of pressure sores. The proper treatment of spasticity is not difficult and can be very beneficial for the overall quality of life. It is one of the more rewarding challenges for the rehabilitation team.

So what is spasticity? It has been defined as *a motor disorder characterized by a velocity-dependent increase in tonic stretch reflexes with exaggerated tendon jerks*. However, this rather bland definition hides the fact that spasticity occurs in a bewildering variety of different forms. It is usually accompanied by various other features of the upper motor neuron syndrome (see next section). It is nearly always accompanied by impairment of voluntary muscle activation. Such impairment will vary, but can include weakness, slowness in building up to maximal power, and clumsiness of voluntary movements. This clumsiness usually results from impaired coordination of the synergistic agonist muscles as well as involving inappropriate restraint or failure of inhibition of the muscles whose action antagonizes the intended movement. The range of voluntary movement that can be achieved is sometimes reduced to just a small number of stereotyped patterns—the so-called *spastic synergies*.

Spasticity is usually demonstrated by imposing a passive movement on a limb and thus inducing involuntary activation of the stretched muscle. Response is usually *velocity dependent* being larger in response to a rapid stretch than a slow stretch. The stretch may trigger a '*spasm*' which is an involuntary and usually self-limiting co-activation of agonist and antagonist muscles of one or more limbs, which can sometimes involve girdle or trunk muscles that are anatomically close to the limbs affected. These spasms are sometimes triggered by cutaneous stimulation. In extensor muscles, especially in the legs, a characteristic pattern is often known as the '*clasp knife response*'. When the muscle is stretched progressively from its shortened position its initial response is the usual velocity-sensitive resistance. However, once a certain length is achieved all resistance dies away and the extensor muscle becomes flaccid only to resume this activation when allowed to shorten. If these features are put together with the other positive and negative features present in the upper motor neuron syndrome then it can be seen that spasticity can cause a bewildering variety of different clinical problems.

At a basic neurophysiological level it has been shown that the alpha motor neurons serving skeletal muscle are hyper-excitable in spasticity and are thus activated by inputs that would not normally provoke any response. In many cases this hyper-excitability is facilitated by the lack of descending inhibitory input from the cortex or higher in the spinal cord. Measures that reduce the activity of the reflex loop from 1a afferent nerve fibres through to the alpha motor neurons can be effective in reducing spasticity. Thus, agents which block sensory inputs such as local anaesthetics or neurolytic drugs, or those which potentiate presynaptic inhibition such as baclofen, have all been shown to reduce the intensity of muscle activation in response to passive stretch. This is a rather simplistic view of neurophysiology of spasticity but nevertheless the over-activity of the afferent/efferent reflex arc at the spinal level provides a model upon which some logical treatment can be based.

Upper motor neuron syndrome

Spasticity is just one of various phenomena that are associated with an upper motor neuron (UMN) lesion. The UMN syndrome is a collection of problems that can occur with any lesion or disturbance of the upper motor neuron pathway. Upper motor neuron lesions cause a variety of both positive and negative features (Table 6.1).

Thus there is a wide range of disturbances in the upper motor neuron syndrome and only one such disturbance is spasticity. In general terms there are many treatment possibilities for the positive features of the UMN syndrome but there are limitations in terms of treatment for the negative features. When treating spasticity the other features of the UMN syndrome that may or may not be present in the individual can have a profound influence on the response to treatment.

Table 6.1 Positive and negative features of UMN lesions

	Muscle weakness
Negative features	Loss of dexterity Fatigability
Positive features	Increased tendon reflexes with radiation Clonus Positive Babinsky sign Spasticity Extensor spasms Flexor spasms Mass reflex Dyssynergic patterns of co-contraction during movement Associated reactions and other dyssynergic and stereotypical spastic patterns

Goals of treatment and outcome measures

The treatment of spasticity, like all rehabilitation processes, should start with the establishment of specific achievable goals and a carefully planned strategy to achieve those goals.

First, does the spasticity need treating at all? Although spasticity is an abnormal neurophysiological event it can still be a positive phenomenon for a given individual. Spasticity in the leg, for example, may serve as a brace to support weight whilst walking or transferring. Arm spasticity can sometimes be useful for assisting in dressing. Some treatments of spasticity can also produce significant side-effects. The oral anti-spastic agents, for example, can induce weakness and fatigue which overall can be more detrimental than leaving the spasticity untreated. In general the goals of treatment of spasticity can be:

- to improve function
- to reduce the risk of unnecessary complications
- to alleviate pain.

Sometimes a goal of the treatment of spasticity is not actually to assist the person with spasticity. Sometimes spasticity can make nursing care particularly difficult. Every time the person is moved a spasm can be induced which can make positioning in bed or a chair or on the toilet extraordinarily difficult. The person themselves may not be particularly bothered by the spasticity or may even be unaware of its presence. A valid reason for treatment is sometimes to ease nursing care in order to assist with the management of hygiene, dressing, and transferring.

Once the goal has been established then a suitable outcome measure needs to be chosen. There are a few documented reliable measures of spasticity but most are really only appropriate in a research setting. The commonest scale is the Modified Ashworth Scale (see Chapter 5 and Table 5.3). There are problems with this scale but nevertheless it is still the most widely used. However, in practical clinical terms it is sometimes valid to use a simple measure that is relevant to the functional goal. If, for example, the aim of treatment is to reduce pain then a simple visual analogue pain scale could be used as an outcome measure. If the aim is to improve walking then a simple 10-m timed walking test may suffice. The outcome measure should be simple and practical and obviously relevant to the stated aim of treatment.

Finally it should be remembered that spasticity is a dynamic phenomenon. It can vary not only according to posture but also according to degree of fatigue, timing of medication, and even the weather. Thus, assessment sometimes needs to be a rather prolonged process with observation of the individual at different times of the day. A quick bedside or outpatient clinic examination is often insufficient and can lead to inappropriate treatment.

Treatment strategies—alleviation of exacerbating factors and positioning

Alleviation of exacerbating factors

There are many external stimuli that can exacerbate and aggravate spasticity. Common causes include:

- Distension or infection of the bladder.
- Constipation.
- Skin irritations, such as in-growing toenails and pressure sores.
- Increased sensory stimuli from external causes, including ill-fitting orthotic appliances, catheter leg bags, and tight clothing or footwear.
- Inappropriate seating or bad positioning in a wheelchair.
- In people who are comatosed or cognitively disturbed then exacerbation of spasticity could be due to underlying abdominal emergency or lower limb fracture.

Sometimes attention to these details can be sufficient to treat the spasticity without other intervention.

Positioning

Probably the most important yet simple treatment is proper seating of the individual. The supine position that is so commonly adopted in the early stages after stroke or brain injury when the person is spending a long time in bed can simply exacerbate extensor spasm by facilitation of the *tonic labyrinthine supine reflex*. Simply sitting the person in a more upright position can avoid this posture and reduce spasticity. In other people, particularly in the early stages after brain injury, an *asymmetric tonic neck reflex* is present. This means if the head is turned to one side then the hip assumes a flexed position in abduction and external rotation whilst the other hip assumes an adducted and internally rotated posture. This is a common cause of later orthopaedic problems, especially in children where it can lead to subluxation of the hip on the adducted side. Awareness of this reflex can prevent the problem. Often periods of *prone lying* with the hips adducted for just 20–30 min can suppress spasticity in the legs for up to 6–8 h. Other postures, such as side lying, sitting, and standing can all be helpful in order to produce stretch on spastic muscles and facilitate use of antagonistic muscle groups.

Treatment strategies—physiotherapy

The most valuable member of the rehabilitation team in terms of treatment of spasticity is the physiotherapist. The physiotherapist has a key role in the following areas:

- Positioning: the importance of positioning has been referred to in the last section and it is usually the physiotherapist who is responsible for appropriate positioning and seating. Sometimes quite complicated seating systems are required to keep the person in a satisfactory and functional position yet at the same time reduce the spasticity. The basic principles of *seating* are that the body should be maintained in a balanced, symmetrical, and stable posture that is both comfortable and maximizes function. Various cushions, foot straps, knee blocks, adductor pommels, lumbar supports, lateral trunk supports, and head and neck support systems have been devised and many are now commercially available.

- Passive stretching: in the early phases after stroke or brain injury or as an on-going process in those with long-standing spasticity passive stretching is vital. Such stretching of spastic muscles, preferably through a full range of movement, can prevent the long term problems of muscle and soft tissue contracture. It is generally recommended that a spastic muscle should be maintained at a position of maximal stretch for around 2h in every 24h. This can be done directly by the physiotherapist. Alternatively the individual can be positioned in a position of maximum stretch in an appropriate seating or standing system or they can be held in a position of stretch by *splinting* or *casting*. Sometimes the use of an orthosis is necessary to stretch the muscle.

- Direct anti-spastic measures: sometimes stretch of the spastic muscle is not possible without the muscle being additionally relaxed. Application of *cold* (e.g. ice packs) or *heat* (such as a warm hydrotherapy pool) are both techniques that can relax the spastic muscle. Another means is *electrical stimulation.*

- Dynamic physiotherapy approaches: there are many schools of physiotherapy which claim that a particular technique has anti-spastic and functional benefits, particularly for the more mobile person. The Bobath technique is widely used, but there are other schools including Proprioceptive Neuromuscular Facilitation and the Brunnstrom technique. There is very little evidence that any particular technique is more efficacious than another and many neurological physiotherapists will now use an eclectic selection of different dynamic approaches to ease spasticity and improve functional gait for a given person.

Treatment strategies—oral medication (i)

Oral medication can bring considerable problems. All anti-spastic drugs can induce weakness and fatigability. Sometimes these side-effects are more troublesome than the original spasticity and all drugs should be used with care and constantly monitored. Available drugs are:

- Diazepam: this was the first anti-spastic agent to be used and probably has an anti-spastic effect by enhancing the action of the inhibiting neurotransmitter GABA (gamma aminobutyric acid). It is certainly an anti-spastic agent but often induces unacceptable weakness and tiredness and is now rarely used.

- Baclofen: this is probably the most widely used oral anti-spastic drug. It is a GABA B receptor agonist that may also work by a presynaptic inhibitory effect on the release of excitatory neurotransmitters such as a glutamate, aspartate and substance P. It has a number of side-effects common to most anti-spastic drugs, including drowsiness, fatigue, and muscle weakness. All these side-effects are dose dependent and unfortunately there is only a narrow therapeutic window between benefit and unacceptable side-effects. Most people need between 40 and 80 mg of baclofen daily in divided doses. The drug should be introduced slowly and withdrawn equally slowly.

- Dantrolene sodium: this is a less useful anti-spastic medication. However, the mode of action is peripheral and it has a direct effect on skeletal muscle. Thus, there is a possibility of having a synergistic effect with other centrally acting agents. It has the usual range of side-effects but in addition can cause hepatoxicity and liver function needs monitoring at regular intervals. Side-effects are reduced if the drug is slowly increased, starting at 25 mg daily and increased over several weeks to a maximum of around 400 mg daily in divided doses.

Treatment strategies—oral medication (ii)

Newer oral anti-spastic drugs

- Tizanidine: tizanidine has fairly recently been introduced into the USA and UK although it is a drug that has been available in some countries for a number of years. The mode of action is largely unknown, but it probably impairs excitatory amino acid release from spinal interneurons, amongst other actions. It seems to be similarly efficacious to baclofen but induces less weakness and is reasonably well tolerated. However, it still has a number of side-effects including dry mouth, fatigue, and dizziness and, like dantrolene sodium, it can be associated with hepatoxicity and liver function needs regular monitoring.

Other anti-spastic drugs

There is a whole range of other anti-spastic agents that have been the subject of studies in the literature. However, few have stood the test of time. The agents that are still available and might be useful include:

- Cannabis: cannabis is likely to be an approved drug in the UK in 2004. There is evidence that it has useful anti-spastic properties as well as being anti-emetic and analgesic. It may turn out to be a useful anti-spastic medication once larger studies have been conducted.
- Clonidine.
- L-dopa.
- Gabapentin: this drug, originally marketed as an anti-convulsant, is showing promising results as an anti-spastic agent as well as being a neuralgic analgesic. It is generally well tolerated and is a useful addition to our armoury of oral anti-spastic agents.

Focal treatment—phenol and botulinum toxin

Most spasticity is focal and just affects one or a few muscle groups. The obvious problem with oral therapy is that it has a generalized systemic effect whereas the aim of treatment is to have an anti-spastic effect only on the spastic muscles. Thus, focal techniques have been developed which avoid the necessity for oral systemic drugs.

Phenol or alcohol nerve blocks

This simple technique involves blockage of a peripheral nerve by injection of phenol or alcohol. Any peripheral nerve that is readily accessible by needle can be blocked. The most useful nerves are:

- Obturator nerve—for adductor spasticity.
- Posterior tibial nerve—for calf spasticity.
- Sciatic nerve—for hamstring spasticity.
- Median, ulnar, or musculocutaneous nerves—for flexor arm spasticity.

The technique is simple and involves injection of the chemical through a needle electrode. The tip of the needle is manipulated to as close as possible to the nerve and its position is confirmed by electrical stimulation. A small volume of phenol or alcohol is then injected down the same needle. This produces an immediate nerve block with relaxation of the supplied muscle. The block will usually last 2–3 months but is sometimes permanent. The technique can be time-consuming and is sometimes uncomfortable. There can be problems with the effect of the block as sometimes a short-term block is needed in recoverable conditions and in such circumstances a long-term block needs to be avoided—but cannot be guaranteed. If a mixed motor/sensory nerve is injected then there can be troublesome sensory side effects including painful dysaesthesiae which can be permanent. However, the overriding advantage is that the technique is simple and cheap and thus can be used in health systems with limited resources.

Botulinum toxin

Botulinum toxin is a potent neurotoxin that blocks the release of acetyl choline from nerve endings. The toxin is available in fixed dose ampoules and will normally require reconstitution in normal saline. The reconstituted solution is then injected directly into the spastic muscle. The toxin will spread within the muscle and over the course of 2–3 days will induce a local relaxation. This anti-spastic effect lasts around 2–3 months before the injection needs repeating. The technique is quick, simple, and effective and there are usually no side-effects. A small number of people can develop a flu-like illness. The main problem is over-relaxation of the muscle inducing unnecessary weakness but with a careful technique this is unusual. However, the toxin is very expensive and is not likely to be used in countries where resources are scarce.

In the long term about 5–10% of people on repeat botulinum toxin injections develop clinical resistance. This is likely to be due to the development of antibodies to the toxin. The most commonly used toxin is type-A toxin (Dysport or Botox). Botulinum toxin type B (Neurobloc or

Myobloc) is now available which in some people can overcome the problem of resistance. However, the type-B toxin does not seem as effective as the type-A toxin and there are a number of troublesome side-effects, including severe dry mouth and pain on injection.

Despite these difficulties botulinum toxin has revolutionized the treatment of spasticity and in many people is now the treatment of choice, after simple measures and physiotherapy, for the management of focal spasticity.

Intrathecal techniques

Intrathecal baclofen

Another way of getting around the problem of oral medication is to inject an anti-spastic agent directly on to the spinal cord. The use of intrathecal baclofen was first described in 1984. This technique involves:

- The implantation of a subcutaneous pump.
- A silastic catheter leading from the pump into the intrathecal space.

The pump is fully programmable and allows the constant infusion of a small dose of baclofen on to the spinal cord. The technique can be useful, particularly in severe and resistant spasticity. It is particularly useful for lower limb spasticity, but intrathecal baclofen will also affect the upper limbs. However, there are disadvantages:

- A surgical procedure is required.
- There is a risk of catheter movement.
- There is a risk of pump failure leading to no dosage or over-dosage of baclofen.

Intrathecal phenol

In some people with very severe spasticity with no motor, sensory, bowel, or bladder function intrathecal phenol can be injected into the lumbar spine to destroy the peripheral nerves and the cauda equina. This works very well in people who are already paraplegic and incontinent but obviously is reserved for people with the most severe problems of spasticity. There is some risk of pressure sores as all sensation below the injected level will be removed.

Surgical and orthopaedic procedures

If spasticity is treated properly in the first instance then it is unusual for a person to require surgery. However, surgery is sometimes required in people with severe or resistant spasticity. It is also required for the management of existing contractures. There are a number of anti-spastic surgical procedures:

- Anterior and posterior rhizotomy—involves section of the spinal reflex arc by cutting the relevant nerves.
- Microsurgical lesions of the dorsal route entry zone (drezotomy)—this is a slightly less invasive technique.
- Percutaneous radiofrequency rhizotomy—an even less invasive technique. It also disrupts the spinal reflex arc.
- Spinal cord and cerebellar stimulation—this is effective but does involve considerable problems with regard to surgery, equipment failure, and expense.

Sometimes surgical repositioning of joints and limbs is necessary for severe spasticity in order to facilitate proper seating, to ease positioning, and to apply orthoses, and reduce the likelihood of further complications. There various orthopaedic interventions but the commonest are:

- Achilles tendon lengthening—for fixed equinus and equinovarus deformities.
- Adductor tenotomies or obturator neurectomies—for severe adductor spasticity.
- Cutting of hamstring tendons or hamstring lengthening procedures—for flexion deformities of the knees.

Upper limb surgery

Surgery in the arm is much more difficult and less successful than in the lower limb, but various tenotomy and tendon lengthening procedures are possible including:

- Lengthening of the biceps and brachioradialis—for elbow flexion deformity.
- Lengthening of the flexor carpi ulnaris and flexor carpi radialis—for wrist flexor spasticity.
- Transfer of the flexor pollicis longus to the radial side of the thumb—for isolated thumb-in-palm deformities.

Shoulder surgery is even more difficult but there are procedures including tenotomy of the pectoralis major, subscapularis, and lattisimus dorsi for severe internal rotation of the shoulder.

This is not a definitive review of surgical techniques for the management of spasticity but gives some idea of potential surgical interventions. However, it is important to emphasize that proper treatment in the early stages of spasticity should mean that surgery is rarely needed.

Continence

Introduction

Neural control of the bladder and bowel extends from the frontal lobes to the sacral cord; bladder dysfunction is extremely common in many neurological diseases and trauma. Incontinence is a major disabling problem, but can often be greatly assisted by fairly simple means. Two major goals exist in treatment:

- management of symptoms, particularly incontinence
- minimization of kidney damage.

Renal failure has been a major cause of mortality, particularly after spinal cord injury, and proper rehabilitation, urological assessment, and follow-up can prevent this, so that renal compromise and death reflect inadequate care nowadays. Faecal incontinence is managed for its devastating impact on socialization rather than its risk to health.

The prevalence of incontinence in neurologically disabled people and in the elderly with multi-organ failure is:

- urinary—generally unknown, but common;
- faecal—considerably less common: it is a feature of autonomic failure, e.g. in diabetes mellitus.

Normal bladder function

The anatomy and physiology are complex (Fig. 7.1). The bladder is composed of detrusor muscle, which allows urine to be collected and the bladder to expand without a rise in pressure until voiding is imminent. The bladder smooth muscle contracts to start voiding and the striated fibres of the external sphincter, which is separately innervated, relax.

Neural innervation

- Autonomic nerve supply. The main nerve supply to the body of the detrusor muscles is from parasympathetic neurons lying in the cord at S2/3/4 level. The bladder, particularly the neck, also receives a supply from the thoracolumbar sympathetic chain. The post-ganglionic sympathetic fibres are adrenergic, whereas the pre-ganglionic sympathetic fibres and parasympathetic fibres are cholinergic. Other neurotransmitters are involved, but this simple classification is useful when considering treatment.

- Somatic nerves. The urethral sphincter has a motor innervation from the discrete Onuf's nucleus at the S2/3/4 level in the cord. This is integrated with the parasympathetic supply, which also arises in this vicinity, and the motor fibres pass into the pudendal nerve, which supplies both the urethral and anal sphincters (Fig. 7.2).

- Sensory nerves. Bladder sensation is mostly conveyed via the pelvic and pudendal nerves to the spinal cord and upwards via the lateral spinothalamic tract. Afferent fibres will synapse in Onuf's nucleus to form a simple spinal reflex as well as also synapsing with the sympathetic chain.

- Pontine micturition centre. This provides a coordinating function regulating long spinal reflexes and receiving modulatory (mainly inhibitory) influences from higher brain centres.

- Higher cortical influence. Pathology of the anteromedial parts of the frontal lobes gives rise to problems in micturition and defaecation, such as urgency, urge incontinence, loss of bladder sensation, and urinary retention. Other frontal lobe lesions produce social disinhibition and voiding at inappropriate times and places, although the voiding mechanism is normal.

1. Frontal micturition area
2. Pontine micturition area
3. Thoracolumbar sympathetic chain
4. Onuf's nucleus
5. Parasympathetic nerves
6. Somatic pudendal nerve
7. Detrusor muscle
8. External urethral sphincter

Fig. 7.1 Neural control of the bladder.

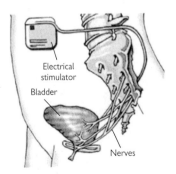

Fig. 7.2 Anterior sacral stimulator (Bradley Scott).

Pathophysiology

Bladder and bowel disorders result from three levels of interruption: suprapontine, suprasacral, and lower motor neuron (Table 7.1).

Bladder detrusor–sphincter dyssynergia

This describes the failure of the sphincter to relax when the detrusor muscle contracts and is due to a spinal cord lesion causing incoordination governing the external sphincter and detrusor muscle of the mechanism. It can give rise to raised intravesical pressure, upper tract dilatation, back pressure on the kidneys, and renal damage. In addition, it can trigger distant problems in spinal cord injured patients with intact sensation with a consequent risk of hypertensive crises. Symptoms result in interrupted bursts of urinary flow between the detrusor forces expelling urine and the sphincter retaining urine.

Table 7.1 Pathophysiology of bladder and bowel disorders

Lesion	Functional change	Disease examples	Outcome
Suprapontine	Frontal lobe disconnection. Periventricular demyelination. Dilatation of lateral ventricle anterior horns	Brain injury. Stroke. MS. Parkinson's disease	Hyper-reflexic bladder contractions. Rarely, urinary retention
Suprasacral	Inhibition from medullary or spinal cord lesion. Descending tract lesions lead to incoordination of external sphincter and detrusor action	Spinal injury or dysfunction, etc.	Hyper-reflexic bladder contractions producing urgency, frequency, urge incontinence. Detrusor-sphincter dyssynergia
Lower motor neuron	S2/3/4 damage gives loss of bladder sensation. Hypotonic bladder with relaxed external sphincter	Lumbar disc prolapse. Trauma. Intraspinal lesions	Urinary retention and leakage. High residual volumes. Stress incontinence

Management of urinary problems

A summary of the management of urinary problems is given in Table 7.2 and Fig. 7.3.

Catheters

Intermittent catheters are safe, but require patient compliance, upper limb functioning and positioning skills for insertion. A small balloon should be employed to reduce nociceptive irritation. In-dwelling catheters should be inserted under aseptic conditions. Complications include leakage, blockage, stone formation, infection, and bladder constriction. Using larger catheters against leakage is erroneous, as they will simply increase detrusor irritability. Anticholinergic medication is useful to suppress detrusor activity. The suprapubic route is preferable in the long term due to better safety and urethral protection profiles.

Surgery

Please refer to a urology text for the indications and description of individual surgical procedures (see Table 7.3). Close working with a urology team is essential part of the rehabilitation team's work.

Table 7.2 Management of urinary problems

Problem	Action	Reason
Impairment of renal function	Investigate (biochemical screen, ultrasound, intravenous urogram (IVU)) and manage medical aspects	Need to preserve renal function for general health and life
Failure of bladder emptying	Assess post-micturition volume by catheter drainage or ultrasound. >100 ml significant	Residual urine stone formation, infection, renal dysfunction
	Involve continence nurse adviser: catheterization—intermittent	Intermittent catheterization carried out by the individual or carer by clean rather than sterile technique using an 8F or 10F catheter. At least twice daily. Best suited for people with functioning sphincters
	Catheterization—in-dwelling	Used when intermittent catheterization is not possible. Size 14F–16F silastic catheter. The suprapubic route is preferable in long-term use because of better safety and urethral protection profiles (see text)
	Sacral nerve stimulation	Fig. 7.2 Control junction
	Treat any urinary infections	Protect renal function and general health
	Urinary retention (rare) due to poor detrusor contraction	Cholinergic, anti-cholinesterase or selective α-1 blocker medication
Detrusor hyper-reflexia	Cystometrogram	Assess intravesical pressure and detrusor hyper-reflexia
	Bladder training	Reduce intravesical pressure
	Anticholinergic medication.	Reduce detrusor activity.
	Botulinum toxin	Intramuscular botulinum toxin has produced good results and lasts about 9 months.
		Injected via cystoscope
	Catheter and condom drainage.	Protection against urinary leaking
	Absorbent pads, napkins, etc.	

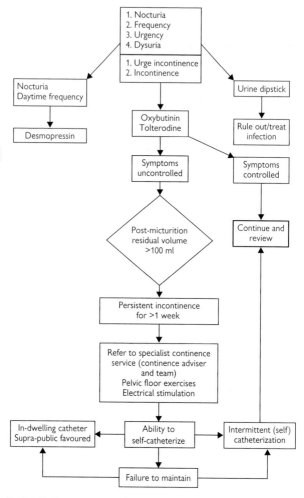

Fig. 7.3 Bladder management pathway.

Table 7.3 Surgical procedures for urinary incontinence

Procedure	Description
Sphincter ablation	Need for this has decreased since the use of botulinum toxin into the detrusor muscle. Sphincterotomy is rare now outside some spinal injuries units
Urinary diversions	Metrofanoff procedure (ileal conduit) allows good bladder control and can change people's lives
Other procedures	Clam cystoplasty. Artificial urethral sphincters and sacral stimulators depend on an intact lower motor neuron. Very effective, but require patient compliance

Sex and sexuality

General issues

Sex and sexuality is the most ignored and least discussed of disability issues. It is not actually known how many people among the disabled population report sexual dysfunction, but figures as high as 72% have been suggested. Professionals are often very embarrassed to talk about the subject and many still have an attitude that it is not a feature that is either worth mentioning or that is relevant to the lives of disabled people. There still persists today a feeling that disabled people should not have sexual feelings. The importance of sex and sexuality and discussing the emotional needs of disabled individuals and their families and carers is an essential part of discovering the whole person whom one is trying to help.

Definitions

- Sexual function, taken outside the context of emotional needs, concentrates on physical function.
- Sexuality includes making relationships, the whole question of self-esteem, personal appearance, and attraction to potential partners and is the very essence of the human spirit. It plays a full part in the lives of not only disabled people but of the general population as well.

The desires and wishes of disabled people for emotional and personal attachments are no different from those of the rest of the population. They are often played down, and it is known that people who have been disabled either from birth or from a very early age have decreased expectations. Their families also have decreased expectations, and it is perhaps not surprising that many disabled people are scared or embarrassed to raise sex and sexuality as an issue. It is therefore important for the doctor or other members of the rehabilitation team to bring up the subject in an open and frank way, so that the whole subject can be discussed freely. There is often a huge relief of emotional frustration once a disabled person can find an appropriate outlet for their feelings. Some psychosexual clinics have been established, but are still relatively uncommon. The teaching of sex and sexuality is now part of the curriculum for specialist trainees in rehabilitation medicine and concentrates on both the psychosocial aspects and the physical function. Various techniques can get round the physical problems and some will be mentioned below. However, the whole idea of a man or woman with a physical disability discussing their sex life with a total stranger fills many with dread.

Common questions are:

- How might they be able to carry out intercourse while having a catheter *in situ*?
- Will they have an episode of incontinence during intercourse; how will they physically get close enough to each other; and how might they relate a relationship to their friends and family?
- How will they deal with the prospect perhaps of pregnancy and parenthood?

Disabled people may well fail initially (just like most of the able-bodied population) but will need to persevere, to learn how to be intimate with their partners without being overwhelmed by failing to match up to their own expectations.

Sexuality

While sex is the act of intimacy, sexuality is the persona of the individual which attracts potential partners. As stated above, disabled young people may be actively hindered in expressing their own sexual feelings. Many men may be impotent and 80 to 90% of such cases are usually psychogenic. With time, relaxation, and confidence, impotence usually resolves, but there are always going to be a few who are going to need help to get over this problem. Again, as stated above, sexual performance need not necessarily be considered as the only yardstick to measure satisfaction in personal relationships. The promotion of quality of life in an open and full relationship may be just as rewarding as the ability to carry out sexual intercourse.

Male sexual function

Impotence tends to be associated with lesions of the spinal cord or cauda equina. Involvement of the autonomic and sensory pathways may give rise to impaired erectile function in males, due to impaired vasocongestion of the corpora cavernosa and spongiosa. The lower the level of the lesion, the more likely that impotence will be organic in nature. Those people with an intact sacral portion of the spinal cord are likely to achieve reflex erection, although this may be inadequate for intercourse. Overall, about half of spinal cord injured men have sufficient erection for intercourse. Sacral anterior stimulator implants can be used to achieve erection, but more commonly men with erectile dysfunction have historically been managed by the use of intracavernosal injections of papaverine. This can give rise to penile fibrosis, but the technique has been successful; it has now been superseded by sildenafil (Viagra). This drug, taken 1 h or so before intercourse, is useful in allowing an appropriate development of an erection in response to a normal emotional stimulation. There is a dose-related response, but most people find that between 25 and 100 mg is sufficient, with 50 mg being the standard dose. It may give rise to coronary insufficiency and care should be taken in people as they get older. It is contraindicated in established coronary artery disease. Prostaglandin E1 (Muse) is again of interest in producing penile rigidity by local stimulation of the glans penis and is therefore recommended for people unable to take sildafenil. The drug is applied with an applicator and an erection may expected within 15 min.

Ejaculatory function is affected more commonly than erectile function in spinal cord injured men. Only 5% of men with a complete upper motor neuron lesion and 18% with a complete lower motor neuron lesion report any persistence of the ability to achieve ejaculation. The treatment may consist of vibration applied to the penis with or without electrical stimulation, using a probe placed in the rectum. This can promote ejaculation by allowing the semen to be collected, but it has to be stated that these techniques are in the management of infertility in spinal cord injured patients rather than in the promotion of the sexual act. Electroejaculation is also possible in the clinic, but again this is for achievement of fertility. All vibration techniques are able to be used at home, but care is required in patients with an injury above the level of D6. Autonomic hyper-reflexia can occur with all its attendant problems. Management of urinary infections is obviously important as such infections will limit already impaired spermatogenesis. Similarly, the older fashioned techniques of sphincterotomy may result in retrograde ejaculation of semen and this procedure is finding less and less favour for many other reasons.

Female fertility

One of the main aspects of sexuality in disabled women is that they may not have received education on contraception. While 75% of men report sexual dysfunction, it is less common in women, at 56%. However, many describe fatigue, diminished sensation, loss of libido, and orgasmic dysfunction. This is particularly evident in those with multiple sclerosis and traumatic brain injury. Hyposexuality is a common change after the latter, although disinhibition and hypersexuality have been reported following a frontal injury.

Pregnancy carries with it increased risks, particularly of pressure sores and sepsis, especially in the urinary tract. Ante-natal care should be carried out in conjunction with a spinal injuries unit. Women with injuries at the D10 level or above are at risk of premature delivery and at D6 and above of autonomic dysreflexia, which is particularly evident as a warning of impending labour. Epidural anaesthesia should be considered as the method of choice for these particular women.

Chapter 9

Eating and swallowing disorders

Introduction

Swallowing disorders are common. Probably about half of people after stroke have a swallowing disorder at some point during the recovery process and problems with swallowing are as common after traumatic brain injury, Parkinson's disease, and in the later stages of multiple sclerosis and motor neuron disease. A whole variety of other neurological problems such as myasthenia gravis and muscular dystrophies, as well as a range of local pathologies, such as mouth and laryngeal cancer, can also cause swallowing difficulties.

Swallowing is essential to maintain nutrition and to deal with saliva. About 1–1.5 l of saliva are produced daily, which requires an awake adult to swallow about once per minute—around 1000 times per day plus the additional swallowing required during eating.

First it is important to recognize that a swallowing problem exists. Sometimes the problem is obvious and the person will volunteer a difficulty with chewing, swallowing, coughing, or spluttering during or soon after eating. However, occasionally the problem is less obvious, particularly in children or those with cognitive impairments. The clues in such individuals may be as follows:

- Recurrent chest infections.
- Weight loss.
- Malnutrition.
- Taking excessive time over food.
- Food residue in the mouth after eating.
- Excessive secretions.
- Wet or hoarse voice after food.
- Sensation of food sticking in the throat.
- Reflux or regurgitation of food or fluid.
- Difficulty breathing.
- Pain when swallowing.
- Laborious chewing.
- Increased throat clearing.
- Post-prandial wheezing.

Thus, there are many clues to eating and swallowing disorders for people who are not able to report difficulties themselves.

The recognition of such disorders is vital, as malnutrition and recurrent pneumonia commonly accompany recurrent swallowing problems. The advent of percutaneous endoscopic gastrostomy (PEG) feeding has now made the management of swallowing disorders much simpler once the diagnosis is made.

Assessment

The clinical assessment of dysphagia is a multidisciplinary process. There are now expert speech and language therapists who specialize in dysphagia management who will work in partnership with the dietician and physician—particularly a radiologist to undertake videofluoroscopic assessments and a surgeon to undertake insertion of PEG feeding tubes.

As in all branches of medicine it is first important to take a thorough clinical history. Not all problems with eating are associated with problems of swallowing. In some people difficulty with behaviour, mood, or cognition can all interfere with or prevent eating. People with a reduced level of alertness may have difficulty eating. After stroke, for example, severe problems of perception or dyspraxia can prevent the individual using plates and cutlery properly. They may not be able to see or recognize food or may be incapable of coordinating the necessary hand and mouth movements to eat and drink. There may be problems cutting up food or difficulty holding a cup because of severe tremor. Problems with receptive language can prevent someone from understanding instructions that 'dinner is ready'. An individual with severe depression may simply not wish to eat. Thus, a swallowing and nutritional assessment cannot be taken out of context from a general assessment of behaviour, mood, cognition, and intellect.

Nutritional assessment
Assessment should be made of the nutritional state. Body weight and height measurements can lead to a calculation of the surface area to weight ratio. Ideal ratios are known. Total body fat can be estimated by skin-fold measurements, such as the biceps, triceps, or iliac sites, and normal parameters are available. An accurate weight record is sometimes the only way to determine whether there is an on-going nutritional or swallowing problem.

Examination of the oral cavity and tongue
The general condition of the mouth, teeth, and the fit of the dentures all need proper examination. There may be:
• Trauma, infection, or structural abnormality in the oral cavity.
• Impaired secretion of the salivary glands.
• Decayed or inadequate dentition or poorly fitting dentures.

All these features will obviously need different treatments in their own right.

Examination of swallowing
A limited amount of information can be obtained from observing a normal swallow. The individual should be alert and seated in an upright and symmetrical position. It is useful for the person to swallow water as well as food with a thick, smooth consistency, such as custard or yoghurt. The examiner should see if the larynx rises to indicate a swallow or if there are clinical signs of swallowing dysfunction such as coughing, spluttering, respiratory distress, or a wet hoarse voice.

There is, however, only one proper way to assess swallowing and that is by use of a *videofluoroscopic swallowing examination*. This will allow assessment of swallowing function during all stages of the swallowing process. In most assessments a number of different food consistencies are given, such as barium liquid, barium mixed with yoghurt, and a barium cookie. The radiologist will screen the chewing and swallowing phases in order to make a diagnosis of the problem. Sometimes various manoeuvres can be tried out during the screening sessions that might improve the individual's swallowing function (see later).

The commonest result of swallowing problems is misdirection of the food or fluids into the airway—known as *penetration*. The passage of food past the vocal cords into the trachea and beyond can cause varying degrees of respiratory discomfort or respiratory compromise. The extent to which inhaled food causes a problem will depend on the amount and frequency of the aspiration as well as the individual's own general condition. Some individuals seem to tolerate aspiration without problems but in most people aspiration is likely to lead to recurrent chest infections and pneumonia.

Finally it is important to note the presence of a *gag reflex* should *never* be taken as a sign of safe oral feeding.

Carer/feeder assessment

Sometimes an apparent eating or swallowing problem is not confirmed on examination and the difficulty is actually not a problem with the disabled person but with the carer or feeder. Time and care in food preparation is often required and considerable effort is sometimes needed in the feeding process. A child with cerebral palsy, for example, can take up to an hour to take an adequate meal. Rushed preparation and inappropriate attention to posture and to the likes and dislikes of the individual can all lead to problems.

Nerve supply

A number of cranial nerves are involved in the swallowing process (see Table 9.1). Normal clinical examination of these cranial nerves is an important part of the overall assessment of someone with swallowing difficulties.

Table 9.1 Cranial nerves involved in the swallowing process

Cranial nerve	Function
V	Muscles of mastication and sensation to the anterior two-thirds of the tongue and buccal cavity
VII	Nerve to supply the orbicularis oris muscle required for lip closure and taste to the anterior two-thirds of the tongue
IX	Taste and sensation to the posterior third of the tongue and buccal cavity and sensation to the tonsils, laryngeal mucosa, and soft palate and involvement of the gag and cough reflexes
X	Similar to IX but also involved with phonation and vocal cord closure in the larynx and sensation and motility of the oesophagus
XII	Movement of the tongue

Normal swallowing mechanism

Swallowing is conveniently divided into four main stages:

- Stage 1—oral preparation. At this stage food is bitten, chewed, and masticated and compressed into a bolus. This phase will clearly rely on proper coordination of the lips, tongue, and jaw and will require an adequate quantity of saliva (Fig. 9.1(1)).
- Stage 2—oral phase. This stage involves the voluntary transfer of the bolus or fluid towards the pharynx. The tongue plays a major part in this process and will move the food bolus upwards and backwards to contact with the hard palate. When the bolus reaches the anterior faucial arch the reflex swallow is initiated (Fig. 9.1(2, 3)).
- Stage 3—pharyngeal phase. This is a reflex stage and is no longer under voluntary control (Fig. 9.1(4, 5)). This stage will involve a number of important muscular actions:
  - Closure of the velopharynx to prevent food and fluid refluxing into the nose.
  - Closure of the larynx to prevent material entering the larynx. This is achieved by laryngeal elevation and anterior movement which also has the effect of stretching and helping to open the cricopharyngeal muscle.
  - Peristalsis of the pharynx in order to help propel the bolus towards the oesophagus.
  - Opening of the cricopharyngeal muscle and passage of the bolus into the oesophagus.
- Stage 4—oesophageal phase. This is again an automatic stage involving passage of the bolus from the relaxed upper oesophageal sphincter at the level of the cricopharyngeal muscle down the oesophagus to enter the stomach through the relaxed gastro-oesophageal/cardiac sphincter (Fig. 9.1(6)).

It is important to emphasize that videofluoroscopy is the only way to obtain an accurate assessment of swallowing and a determination of the part of the swallowing process that is at fault.

Video recording is possible, which allows a more detailed analysis of the rapid automatic swallowing phases.

Fig. 9.1 The four stages of swallowing: (1) oral preparatory stage; (2, 3) oral stage; (4, 5) pharyngeal stage; (6) oesophageal stage.

Management of swallowing problems

As with all parts of the rehabilitation process it is important that any treatment intervention is accurately monitored. Repeat videofluoroscopy may be used, but obviously there are limits to the number of times a videofluoroscopy can be repeated. Thus other less direct measures of monitoring are useful, such as regular monitoring of the weight. In particular calculation of the body mass index (BMI) is useful. This is calculated as the weight (in kg) divided by the height (in metres) squared. It is also useful to maintain an accurate diet history. This can include the details of the food and liquid intake as well as the consistency of the food, the number of times the individual coughs or splutters on food during a typical meal, and length of time taken to complete the meal, etc.

Next it is necessary to calculate energy and protein requirements so that the necessary dietary intake can be calculated. At this point involvement of a dietician becomes essential.

Modifying the oral diet

The videofluoroscopy may well have indicated the type of food consistency that is best tolerated. It is often the case that thin fluids, such as soup, or crumbling foods, such as biscuits, are best avoided. Usually smooth, semi-solids are best, which in turn requires thickened fluids or a pureed or soft diet. Once again advice from a dietician is necessary as such diets can be bland and disliked by the individual.

The videofluoroscopy may have indicated other possible compensatory strategies. Some general guidelines would include:

- Posture—variations to head and neck posture can sometimes alleviate a swallowing disorder and in any case, if at all possible, the head and neck should be upright and symmetrical.
- Learning to relax and not to talk during eating can be helpful.
- It is often useful to develop a feeding regime that involves small amounts of food in the mouth with a quite clear deliberate chewing phase leading to a purposeful swallow.
- Generally several small meals a day are preferable to two or three big meals both from the point of view of the swallowing and to eliminate problems with fatigue—both in the disabled person and the carer.
- There is some evidence that exercises can improve oral motor control, strength, and range of movement and bolus control.
- There are some specific techniques for a delayed swallowing reflex. In such people the reflex is triggered too late to prevent some aspiration. In some cases stroking of the faucial arches with a cold laryngeal mirror prior to eating seems to trigger a reflex more effectively. Occasionally sucking on ice can have a similar effect.

Nutritional supplements

Nutritional supplements should be considered as soon as there is evidence that the dietary intake alone is insufficient. There is now a wide range of oral nutritional supplements. These are generally protein and energy dense and are also prescribable in a variety of flavours. There are also high-energy snacks, meals, and drinks that can supplement an inadequate diet.

Artificial nutritional support

When oral nutrition is contra-indicated because of the risk of aspiration or is inadequate to meet nutritional requirements then some form of non-oral feeding becomes necessary. There are basically two non-oral routes—nasogastric feeding and gastrostomy feeding.

Nasogastric feeding

Nasogastric feeding is quick to initiate and is often used in the early days after an acute event, such as a stroke or brain injury when the individual is unable to take any or little oral nutrition. There are now highly durable fine-bore polyurethane tubes that are easy to insert and reasonably comfortable to have *in situ* for a few days. However, there are significant problems with nasogastric feeding. Many people find the tube uncomfortable. The tubes often need replacement and re-intubation can be upsetting as well as a potential cause of nasal trauma. Other disadvantages include blocking of the tube, displacement of the tube, and indeed the nasogastric tube itself might further impair a defective swallowing mechanism.

Percutaneous endoscopic gastrostomy

In recent years percutaneous endoscopic gastrostomy (PEG) feeding has gained wider acceptance as a quick and safe alternative to a surgical gastrostomy. There is no need for general anaesthesia and insertion of the tube is a simple procedure just requiring a local anaesthetic and sometimes a short-term intravenous sedative. There is a very low complication rate of less than 1%. Tubes can be placed under radiological direction or more commonly by assistance with an endoscope. The tubes are well tolerated and there is less risk of tubes becoming blocked or being dislodged.

Tube feeds can be administered either by bolus or by continuous pump. Sometimes overnight feeding via a pump is useful in supplementing an inadequate oral intake. However, for those who need most or all of their nutrition through the tube then bolus feeding is generally best as this has the advantage that the patient is free to be more mobile for large parts of the day. Usually boluses are administered at 4–6 h or indeed at normal mealtimes. Usually people can tolerate 200–400 ml of a feed at a time which will require just three to four feeds per day. Liquid medication can also be given down the tube.

Problems

Other than problems with the tube itself, such as blockage and dislodging, there are a number of common problems such as diarrhoea, abdominal pain, abdominal distension, gastric reflux, and vomiting. Sometimes it can be quite a long process to adjust the feeding regime to reduce such symptoms to a minimum.

However, PEG feeding is usually easy and safe and is now widely practised for many people both in the short term following a recoverable condition, such as stroke or brain injury, or in the long term for those with permanent swallowing disorders, such as those with multiple sclerosis or motor neuron disease.

Communication

Introduction and referral

Communication encompasses speech, non-verbal communication and special senses (the ability to hear and to see) and is reliant on normal cognitive function. Speech and language therapists have a major role to play in the assessment of communication and in the treatment of its disorders, but the whole rehabilitation team has to be skilled in recognizing ways to communicate with patients. People with communication disorders are often frequently poorly appreciated and feel that it is the world at large that has the problem. Those with pure motor speech deficits on the other hand, usually understand that they have a problem and become immensely frustrated by it.

Assessment

Those whose communication interferes with their participation in society require an assessment from a speech and language therapist. Assessment may take quite a long time, even in skilled hands, and other professionals simply do not have the time or the expertise to develop a thorough appreciation of the problems. Care should be given to ensuring that at the time of referral the patient can actually cope with and understand the assessment process. Speech and language therapists are concerned with all aspects of communication in terms of improving personal communication skills in general, including non-verbal communication, and can pass on that advice to the rest of the rehabilitation team. They can thus provide other team members and families with a consistent approach to patients to achieve an appropriate response or reply in order to reduce the frustration to a minimum.

Speech and language disorders

Disorders of speech

- Speech or articulation depends on normal musculature. Loss of neuromuscular control of the structures involved in articulation results in slurring of speech, *dysarthric speech*.
- Tone and quality are affected by damage to the tongue, the lips, the palate, the vocal cords, and lungs, e.g. in the hypernasal sound of cleft palate.
- Damage to articulation can occur following resuscitation after a stroke or traumatic brain injury.
- *Anarthria* is used to describe complete loss of speech due to impairment of neuromuscular control.

Disorders of language

Dysphasia is characterized by four elements:
- Expression (motor).
- Comprehension (receptive).
- Reading.
- Writing.

The causes are a lesion affecting the dominant hemisphere in the parietal and temporal areas. Reading and writing may also be affected, but receptive involvement suggests a more extensive lesion. Global dysphasia suggests impairment of all aspects of language and the patient may only be able to make unintelligible grunting sounds.

Disorders of fluency

Stammering or *stuttering* result from hesitations and blocking of speech and tend to be less common in adults. Chronic neurological disease (spinal cord injury and multiple sclerosis in particular) can produce intercostal and diaphragmatic muscle weakness, which reduces breath control and thus fluency.

Disorders of voice

Dysphonia may be organic or psychological. Polyps, nodules, and oedema of the vocal cords cause abnormal stresses and tensions and are commonly found in singers. Although speech is usually intelligible, it is quite embarrassing for people as it may affect the ability of people to regain work. Such problems may arise, for example, from local laryngeal damage in surgery.

Commonly associated diseases

Stroke
About 15% of stroke sufferers will have a significant dysphasia. Non-dominant parietal lobe lesions in stroke may give a transient dysarthria, which usually recovers well, but there may also be a loss of non-verbal communication. Disorders of expression after stroke are due to motor lesions in the postero-superior temporal and frontal lobe. Disorders of comprehension are due to sensory lesions of the postero-inferior temporal lobe.

Traumatic brain injury
Both dysphasia and dysarthria are seen, but often resolve quite quickly in contrast to the situation in stroke patients. The main communication difficulties lie in non-verbal communication and cognitive deficits, and the speech and language therapist works with the rest of the rehabilitation team to find a consistent way to approach and communicate with the disabled individual.

Multiple sclerosis
Spastic and ataxic dysarthria may both occur with disease progression from difficulties around the tongue and mouth. As a result, feeding difficulties may occur.

Other chronic neurological diseases
Parkinson's disease, motor neuron disease, and myasthenia gravis all produce dysarthrias and dysphonias and patients with Parkinson's disease classically become quieter as the disease progresses. The on–off periods of disease control affect speech greatly and very often one can judge symptom control on speech alone.

Cerebral palsy
Communication is a major feature of assessment. Dysarthria and dysphonia are common, but language disorders are less common and are usually associated with learning disabilities. Signing systems such as hand signs, Makaton, or Bliss signs can improve communication and the input of a speech and language therapist is very important here.

Communication aids

Communication aids may be useful substitutes for verbal communication and may transform a person's life (see Table 10.1). They are indicated for severe dysarthria and expressive dysphasia, yet may be quite simple. They tend to be less helpful where there is a receptive disorder. Users require considerable motivation, which rules out their use in some people with cognitive or learning difficulties.

Table 10.1 Types of communication aid

Type of aid	Description
Direct select	Uses part of a body to indicate a symbol, e.g. Canon communication aid, a small hand-held method of typing words for communication. The moderately intelligent person may prefer to use a word board, which points to letters, and some become very adept at writing out words
Scanning	This method is chosen for people with very severe physical disabilities and a series of options comes up on a screen. The user can then point or signal the correct choice
Encoding	Uses a key symbol for the use of phrases, so pressing a certain symbol on the keyboard will produce a pre-set phrase and allow more fluent communication. May be used by cognitively intact people who wish to use a relatively large vocabulary. Even though it may be limited shortly after the stroke, encoding methods are ambitious and can be combined with direct selection, scanning, and environmental control equipment

Patient follow-up

Follow-up over many months and even years is essential, as recovery is slow. Users of communication aids must be checked to make certain that they are using them correctly and that the aid is valuable to them in their everyday lives rather than just for therapy. Many find them vital for quality of life, but many also give them up because they can use non-verbal communication better to communicate with their friends and family. More extensive communication aids can be obtained from regional centres, such as the Access to Communication Technology.

Chapter 11

Other physical problems

This chapter will include some of the many physically disabling conditions which do not conveniently fit into either diagnosis- or impairment-based classifications, such as pressure sores, contractures, pain within the context of physical disability, and the chronic fatigue syndrome (ME, fibromyalgia, etc.).

Pressure sores

Definition
Pressure sores are defined as an area of erythema under the skin, which may progress to ulceration and subcutaneous tissue necrosis as a result of ischaemia due to unrelieved pressure.

Features
Pressure sores cause significant mortality and morbidity. Ninety-five per cent of them are totally preventable and result in an immense cost the the National Health Service. Three to 11% of all patients admitted to hospital develop a pressure sore. Pressure sores are caused by ischaemia and by damage to subcutaneous blood vessels and are characterized initially by persistent skin erythema where pressure from friction forces injures blood vessels in the skin. This results in ischaemia, cell necrosis, and superficial ulceration. Deeper structures may be affected by shear forces occurring in the neighbourhood of bony prominences, which give rise to more extensive subcutaneous destruction. The necrotic tissue invariably becomes infected, causing inflammation of surrounding tissues and systemic toxicity. Maceration of the skin by sweat and urine reduces its tensile strength and the elderly are at special risk because ageing decreases the skin's tolerance to stress and increases the likelihood of breakdown.

Clinical features and staging
- Stage 1. Discoloration of intact skin including non-blanchable erythema or loss of epidermis. Starts at the surface and progresses inwards.
- Stage 2. Partial skin loss involving the epidermis and dermis. Heals within weeks.
- Stage 3. Full-thickness skin loss extending to subcutaneous tissues. Starts deep and causes skin necrosis from below. Takes months to heal.
- Stage 4. Full-thickness skin loss with extensive destruction involving muscle and bone and other deep structures with tissue necrosis.

Who is at risk?
Table 11.1 shows the main risk factors for the development of pressure sores.

Pressure sore management
Management of pressure sores is described in Table 11.2.

Table 11.1 Risk factors associated with the development of pressure sores

Immobility	Neurological disease, especially tetra/paraplegia
	Obesity
	Coma/confusion
Sensory loss	Severe physical disease
	Weight loss
	Low albumin
	Low vitamin C
Deformity	Producing abnormal loads
	Fractures
	Faecal and urinary incontinence
Prevention	Use of Norton or Waterlow scale
	Education of 'At risk' patients
	Management of deformities and 2–3 hourly turning
	Seating, cushions and mattresses

Norton, D. (1961). *Nursing Times* **57**:695–6. Waterlow, J. (1985). *Nursing Times* **81**:49–55.

Table 11.2 Management of pressure sores

Physical measures	Relief of pressure is the most important factor. Debridement of necrotic tissue, which can be done on the ward in insensate patients, speeds up the healing process
General health	A good diet containing protein and vitamin C is essential. Haematinics to treat anaemia. Transfusion if haematinics cannot maintain Hb of 10 g/dl. Treatment of constipation/faecal loading. Prevention of urinary/faecal incontinence
Topical treatments	Semi-permeable films to cover ulcers and soothe the skin. Antiseptic agents to reduce infection. Alginate dressings/hydrocolloid/hydrogel systems to absorb exudate. Enzymes, hydrocolloid and hydrogel systems to remove slough. Agents to promote granulation tissue
Infection	Antibiotics necessary for deep sores and for underlying bone infection
Surgery (adjunct to conservative therapy only)	Primary repair. Formal plastic and reconstructive surgery to provide skin and muscle flaps for weight-bearing areas (buttock, sacrum, trochanters), as a graft will often not survive the stresses and strains

Contractures

Definition

Contracture is restriction of limb movement leading to loss of function (dexterity, mobility, etc.).

Features

Tendon and joint contracture occur in prolonged immobility, due to either neurological or musculoskeletal pathology. Muscle and tendon shortening or joint capsule restriction occur leading to fibrosis and loss of range of movement across articulations and limbs. The process may start as a result of pain in a limb, joint disease, spasticity, or simple poor positioning. As a result, much time must be spent in stretching the limbs in order to reverse the process and contractures lead to severe problems, such as pain, problems with perineal hygiene, inability to place the foot flat on the ground, loss of dexterity, and notably poor self-esteem and mood changes.

Treatment

Treatment is often difficult and often painful, but where contractures are established, serial splinting and/or surgery should be considered:

- Splinting: The limb is stretched and a resin cast is applied, which is left for 7 to 10 days and then removed. The limb is then stretched further and a new cast is applied. Very often, back slabs or univalved cylinders are used to facilitate inspection of the limb and allow physiotherapy.
- Surgery: Where return of limb function is not possible, as in patients with severe hemiplegia or paraplegia, tenotomy or arthrotomy operations may be needed to allow tissue release and further stretching is applied.

Chronic pain

Conditions commonly associated with chronic pain include:
- Chronic musculoskeletal pain, e.g. neck and back pain.
- Occupational upper limb disorders.
- Degenerative joint disease.
- Reflex sympathetic dystrophy (Sudek's atrophy).

Central pain syndromes

Thalamic pain following stroke or traumatic brain injury is disabling and can lead to dysaesthesia or an awareness of abnormal sensation in the affected area of the body, very often down one side. Disordered function of the spinathalamocortical pathway, which is responsible for pain and temperature, is thought to be the cause. Patients can often experience more than one type of pain. Movement, touch, or cold, especially a cold breeze, can often bring on the pain.

Management should start with anti-convulsants (in particular gabapentin, carbamazepine, or sodium valproate). If these are no help, anti-depressant medication, muscle relaxants and even chlorpromazine can be tried. None of these has been validated for this purpose and none is routinely successful.

Reflex neurovascular dystrophy/reflex sympathetic dystrophy/Sudek's atrophy

This is a group of disorders in which an injury or insult proximally can lead to pain distally in the limb. This pain is continuous in nature and is accompanied by hyperalgesia and allodynia. Local abnormal sympathetic activity is observed, with changes in temperature and colour of the limb and abnormal sweating. The affected part becomes cold and pale and muscles become wasted. Contractures and osteopenia appear, giving the name of Sudek's atrophy. Sympathetic blockade is the treatment of choice, which should be combined with active exercise and physiotherapy. Other measures for chronic pain relief, such as anti-depressant medication, may be required.

Management of pain

A thorough assessment of the patient and carer is required. Where patients have been complaining of pain for years from degenerative disease, further medical intervention may be inappropriate and this should be clearly communicated. However, painful exacerbations need to be treated with effective medication and mild, but active, exercise. Patients should be responsible for their own management and should seek medical assistance only when initial measures have failed. Successful management is critically dependent on finding a regimen of treatment which will help the patient. A combined approach involving physical exercise, medication, and other therapies is required for most patients.

Physical treatments and exercise

Prolonged physiotherapy for people with chronic pain increases dependence on health professionals, and patients should be taught an exercise programme that encompasses general exercise to improve fitness, specific exercises to protect the affected part of the body, and should be given information on how to deal with painful exacerbations. Manipulation and mobilization may be useful for this and for reducing muscle spasm and pain in acute situations, but there is no evidence that they or other treatments alter the natural history of chronic pain.

Transcutaneous nerve stimulation (TENS) or acupuncture are effective in reducing pain and can be used in combination with other treatments. They require suitable education to ensure their efficacy. Splints, corsets, and braces can be helpful for acute exacerbations, but long-term use leads to disuse muscle atrophy and should be avoided.

Medication

A number of medications are available; these are detailed in Table 11.3.

Table 11.3 Medications for chronic pain

Centrally acting analgesics	Start with simple medication and increase the dose and the potency of opioid analgesics. Narcotic analgesics suppress natural endorphin production and can be quite dependent. They thus have no real place in the management of chronic pain
Anti-depressants	Tricyclics have been shown as most useful in treating anxiety and depression in chronic pain and probably have a synergistic action with analgesics. They should be used for periods of 3 to 6 months as shorter periods of time are often ineffective. Both tricyclic anti-depressants and selective serotonin re-uptake inhibitors (SSRIs) have an equal impact on pain relief, although some examples in these groups have a better action than others. Paroxetine tends to be more helpful in this situation than other SSRIs for its greater anxiolytic action. Amitriptyline and dothiepin are useful in inducing sleep when taken at night, allowing a reasonable period of rest for the patient to be more resilient to cope with the following day
Muscle relaxants	These have little role in the treatment of chronic pain. Baclofen and dantrolene sodium are sometimes used for their anti-spasm qualities. Associated with considerable side-effects and dependence and should probably not be used. Long-term use not recommended

Chronic pain (*continued*)

Specific injections
Table 11.4 shows specific injections which may be of use.

Cognitive behavioural therapy
Cognitive behavioural therapy involves developing certain behavioural characteristics to try to normalize activities in chronic pain. Patients encouraged to attempt certain key tasks every day and follows this up with rest and evaluation of the level of pain. It has had an effect in many patients and the aim is to develop a coping strategy to enable participation in day-to-day activities. Time is of the essence here and consistency of approach results in a better response.

Table 11.4 Injections for use in the management of chronic pain

Local injections	Corticosteroids into joints can be helpful in reducing active synovitis, even in the absence of overt inflammation
Local nerve blocks	Relieve pain in a multitude of conditions ranging from soft tissue problems to intractable pain from osteoarthritis, e.g. suprascapular nerve blocks for intractable shoulder pain. Regional sympathetic blockade is used for many conditions, ranging from inflammatory joint disease and osteoarthritis to reflex neurovascular dystrophy. Although the effects are sometimes short-lived, the procedure is relatively straightforward. Even simpler is guanethidine blockade of distal limbs, using 20 mg of guanethidine intravenously in a cuffed limb
Epidural injections	Useful for acute and acute intermittent relief of limb pain. Long-term relief not demonstrated in chronic settings
Facet joint injection	Used in the facet joint syndrome and in lumbar spondylosis, although the evidence does not tend to support this in patient populations. It is probably of value in very specific patients, in whom there is referred pain and localized tenderness over one specific joint. Can allow relief of pain for several weeks, if not months

Chronic fatigue syndrome/fibromyalgia

This is a group of disorders in which there are symptom complexes of widespread musculoskeletal pain, hyperalgesia, tenderness at specific sites, severe fatiguability, and functional disturbance at many levels. The ME syndrome and fibromyalgia have been categorized together under chronic fatigue syndrome. The symptoms and disability caused by this condition are real and are not fabricated or imagined (Table 11.5). The associated disability is functional rather than pathological and the tenderness and associated sleep disturbance are characteristic. This can be reproduced by selective deprivation of non-REM sleep and appears to be universally present in these patients.

Common symptoms of fibromyalgia

- Pain: predominantly of the neck and back aggravated by stress and by cold. Generalized morning stiffness following activity, generalized pain, poor response to analgesics.
- Fatigue: follows even minimal exertion and may be severe.
- Others: subjective limb swelling, paraesthesiae, dysaesthesia of hands and feet, poor sleep, poor concentration, low mood, irritability, weakness, headache, often occipital or bifrontal, diffuse abdominal pain, variable bowel habit, urgency of micturition.

Fibromyalgia is classified as primary and secondary to identified pathology, e.g. osteoarthritis. It is a diagnosed by exclusion of other conditions (e.g. joint and muscle disease, hypothyroidism, systemic lupus erythematosus, hyperparathyroidism, osteomalacia). Patients are often anxious (about underlying pathology, such as cancer or multiple sclerosis) or depressed and women are more commonly affected than men.

Management

It is important to reassure patients that they have a genuine condition and it is not due to their imagination. Nor are they attempting to deceive either the professionals or their families. There is often a considerable element of anxiety among both patients and their families and an overconcerned partner can often generate the problems. Treatment combines medication (tricyclic or selective serotonin re-uptake inhibitor (SSRI) antidepressants) with gentle exercise and cognitive behavioural programmes. These aim to get patients to accept responsibility for their pain and their disability and to increase their belief in their own ability to control pain and to improve energy levels. Even though the pain may still cause problems, the patient eventually becomes more able to increase their social, leisure, and occupational activities.

Prognosis

The prognosis in chronic fatigue syndrome and fibromyalgia is not particularly good. Some self-help groups have been set up and there is a concern that while patients themselves may be helped to understand their problems, the group will contain elements who perpetuate the sick role rather than the benefits of rehabilitation.

Table 11.5 Classification of chronic fatigue disorders

Principal presenting symptom	Diagnostic label
Locomotor pain	Fibrositis, pain amplification syndrome, fibromyalgia
Fatigue	ME syndrome, chronic fatigue syndrome
Headache	Tension headache
Abdominal pain, bowel disturbance	Irritable bowel syndrome

Chapter 12

Technical aids and assistive technology

Introduction

- *Technical aids* cover all equipment for disabled people, whether for use in the home, at work, or in the community at large. They range from simple devices in the kitchen or bathroom, to hoists, stair-lifts, and any item which may improve the standard of living for a disabled person. Some are used personally by the disabled person, whereas others are designed to be operated by carers. Occupational therapists have particular skills in this field and equipment can be viewed and inspected in disabled living centres (contact information through the Disabled Living Foundation). Care equipment helps disabled people, but is also designed to protect their carers from injury, e.g. hoists protect carers from back pain.
- *Assistive technology* encompasses any technical equipment to improve participation and independence among disabled people. It covers simple technical aids and any device (electronic or other) which the disabled person may operate within their home or outdoors. Communication aids are dealt with in Chapter 10.

Wheelchairs

Wheelchairs can be obtained through the National Health Service for people with long-term needs, or can be bought privately. Disabled people have identified specific needs and may require more than one wheelchair—for work, at college, and at home—and services therefore have to be flexible and sensitive to these needs.

Considerations in wheelchair prescription are:
- Diagnosis—affects usage of the chair, the need for review and on the speed of delivery, e.g. in motor neuron disease. Presence of complicating factors, e.g. spasticity.
- Frequency of the chair's use.
- Where will the chair be used? Outdoors? Indoors? Both? Local environmental factors.
- Transfers in and out of the chair—unaided, standing, sideways, assisted by carer, transfer boards etc. Should arm rests be removable to allow sideways transfer?
- Transportation of chair.
- Needs of the carer.
- Seating—need for cushion, special seating or complex seating system, activities in the chair, other factors, e.g. incontinence.

Types of wheelchair
- Push-chair/buggy: for disabled children—similar features to those found for young able-bodied children. Need to be supportive, but easy to use and should be able to fold away.
- Manual self-propelled: 9-series wheelchairs—same sizes as 8 series, but have four small wheels.
- Attendant-propelled: 8L standard 16 inch seat (seat widths available up to 20 inches); 8BL—15 inch by 16 inch seat.
- Powered: for indoor and indoor/outdoor use.

Many models and variations are now available. Attachments include trunk supports, altered armrests, tilting backrests, head supports, and adjustable footrests. More sporty wheelchairs are also now available through NHS provision, which have a greater 'street credibility' amongst the young. Light-weight wheelchairs sacrifice stability for low weight. They thus have to have a rigid frame, which prevents them folding. Powered chairs also do not usually fold. Tetraplegics above the level of C5 may require an electric wheelchair. They are controlled by a joystick on a control box, but some patients may need a chin control, a blow and suck control, a head control, or even a photo-electric cell.

Getting a wheelchair is usually through a loan system, but some patients may use a voucher scheme, which covers their equipment up to a certain financial allowance. They can add to this through their own means.

Special seating

Special seating is that component of a seating system, in either a static chair or a wheelchair, which is specifically prescribed for disabled people to accommodate or control any postural difficulties or to manage problems that may arise from abnormal pressures due to deformity.

Definitions for special seating criteria

- *Mild disability*: Good head control. Good to fair trunk control. May be unstable when sitting unsupported. Good functional ability with minimal support on a stable base.
- *Moderate disability*: Good head control but poor trunk control. Unable to sit in a stable position without support. Limited hand control when sitting in a stable position.
- *Severe disability*: Poor head and trunk control. Unable to sit without support. Limited upper limb function. Spinal curvature and joint contractures.
- *Static support*: Fixed skeletal deformity and pressure problems. Maintains function and prevent deformities from worsening.
- *Dynamic support*: For weakness and motor impairment. Enhances function.

Aims of special seating systems

- To achieve stability and balance.
- To reduce the effort to maintain posture.
- To prevent or delay the onset or worsening of deformities.
- To optimize function.
- To provide comfort.
- To allow distribution of load to provide maximal pressure relief.
- To decrease cardiorespiratory burden through functional support.

The seating system depends on the severity of the disability, the abilities and requirements of the disabled person, the ability and needs of carers, and other environmental factors. Many systems are designed for children with multiple disabilities, including learning difficulties, who may have fixed deformities as a result of poor positioning in early life. An appropriate seating system can improve a person's lifestyle and self-esteem.

A good seating system therefore should aim to:

- Enable good positioning for comfortable sitting, feeding, swallowing, and communication.
- Encourage bladder and bowel drainage and function.
- Provide good eye contact.
- Support the trunk to decrease the effort of breathing.
- Provide comfort.
- Be practical for the carer.

Organization of services

Special seating systems are expensive and, in the context of health-care constraints, cannot be freely available unless there is a clinical need. Simpler seating systems are prescribed by local wheelchair services, but more complex equipment is provided by regional centres. The expertise there, from rehabilitation engineers and specialized rehabilitationists and therapists, ensures a more cost-effective service provision.

Footwear and orthoses

Orthoses are devices worn outside the body which support and aid the function of that part. All doctors and therapists acquire a basic training in orthotics at both undergraduate and postgraduate level, in order to understand their potential value. As with other technical assistance, the decision to use an orthosis should be made after team discussion. The team should include a doctor, a therapist, nursing staff, and orthotists and each orthosis should be prescribed with a specific aim. Both the orthotist and the patient should have a thorough knowledge of what the orthosis is attempting to do. If a device is not worn, then the whole process fails and the technical merits of the appliance serve no useful purpose. The team should thus estimate the patient's compliance and education is an important feature.

Types of orthoses
- Footwear: insoles, shoe modifications, bespoke shoes.
- Supports: collars, lumbar supports/belts, epicondylitis clasps.
- Splints: static/resting (prevents movement and supports joints) or working/lively (helps to increase limb function.

Footwear
Foot pain is common and may be due to joint disease or to nerve injury from unsupported weight-bearing structures. Prevention of subtalar subluxation is important in early joint disease in order to prevent pain distally, and the wearing of good footwear is a cheap and effective way to help with this. Many doctors do not realize how the prescription of comfortable shoes can transform the lives of people with painful feet. The development of depth shoes has increased the range available and there is now less need for individually made (bespoke) surgical shoes.
- Insoles:
  - *Medial longitudinal arch supports*: used for simple flat feet, for lateral plantar nerve compression, and for the prevention of subtalar valgus subluxation, as found in rheumatoid and osteoarthritis.
  - *Metatarsal domes*: transfer weight away from the metatarsal heads to the metatarsal shafts to relieve the pain from metatarso-phalangeal joint disease and subluxation. A larger size of shoe may be needed to prevent callosities on the dorsum of the toes and plastazote temporary domes should first be fitted to test their efficacy.
  - *Heel insoles*: for traumatic heel and leg pain and plantar fasciitis. New materials using shock-absorbing pads are useful in preventing heel pain, e.g. Sorbothane and Viscolast.
- Modified shoes:
  - *Shoe raises*: these are used to correct unequal leg lengths. The same leg length is not required to achieve a normal swing phase in walking and raising the sole by half the difference in leg length works. Differences of less than 1 cm are probably not worth correcting in this way.
  - *Depth shoes*: these are enhanced footwear for people with deformed feet. They are lightweight with a non-slip sole and have a wide opening to allow easy fitting. They are fairly cheap to produce

and cater for most deformities, and sufficient space is available to fit an insole. However, this should be checked first.

- *Bespoke shoes*: individually designed to fit people with difficult feet, and can fulfil a variety of functions from tough working shoes to comfortable lightweight items. They are expensive to make and casts of the foot are made before the final shoe is manufactured. The lengthy time taken in fitting contributes to their high cost.

Supports

- *Collars*: support the neck and reduce pain, but do not truly prevent movement. For really effective immobilization of the head, skull or halo traction should be used. They reduce muscle spasm in the first few days following neck injury and patients with rheumatoid disease should be fitted with one prior to intubation for an anaesthetic.
- *Corsets*: the commonest indication is an acute lumbar disc protrusion with muscle spasm and support for the anterior abdominal wall. Polythene jackets are used with variable success for the pain of osteoporotic vertebral collapse and to prevent the effects on respiration of increasing truncal weakness as seen in muscular dystrophies etc.
- *Epicondylitis clasps*: worn on the proximal forearm to decrease the load on the extensor and flexor muscle origins and tennis and golfer's elbow respectively, they transfer the effective origin point of the muscle to a point under the clasp through a tight grip over the muscle's belly and allow work or the playing of games.

Splints

The functions of splints are to:
- Stabilize joints.
- Reduce pain and inflammation through immobilization.
- Place the limb in the best functional position.
- Protect joints, leading to confident usage.
- Prevent or reduce further deformity.

Serial splinting is used to increase the range of joint movement to reduce joint or tendon limb contracture. It will reduce even very large contractures when accompanied by active physical treatment. The limb is straightened to a comfortable maximum and the splint is applied. The splint is then changed every 7 to 10 days to allow a straighter cast to be applied until the objective is achieved.

There are a number of types of splint:
- *Resting splints* immobilize the affected part of the limb. They are often used at night to rest joints. Help may be required to apply and remove them, particularly if they are bilateral. *Example*: a paddle splint for the wrist and hand for patients with rheumatoid arthritis. Made of orthoplast and used to relieve acutely inflamed joints and useful as a night resting splint; the wrist should be held in 10° of extension when the splint is applied.
- *Working or lively splints* allow a limb to work in some functional way and may incorporate a moving part, either free-moving or against resistance. Stabilizing one joint may result in better functional use of the whole limb. *Example*: hand splint in radial nerve injury.

Footwear and orthoses (*continued*)

- Working wrist splints: the Futuro wrist splint is probably the best known in the UK. There is a metal bar on the volar surface, resting the wrist, but full use of the hand is allowed. The splint is used in carpal tunnel syndrome and in inflammatory arthritis. It is also prescribed in people with repetitive strain disorder, but its use here is probably unwise. An individually made orthoplast or polythene splint may be necessary if the wrist is deformed.
- Working hand splints: indicated, for example, for extensor tendon rupture to preserve function. An opponens splint is used for a painful first carpo-metacarpal joint in osteoarthritis.
- *Knee splints* stabilize knees with collateral ligament or cruciate ligament dysfunction (Table 12.1).
- *Ankle/foot orthoses*: indicated for foot drop following lateral popliteal nerve palsy, L5 nerve root compression, and stroke. Supports ankle and subtalar joint instability and may incorporate insole corrections. Made of lightweight ortholon, which is not particularly strong and can crack. A leg iron caliper, fixed to the heel of the shoe from a strap at the upper calf, may then be required.

How to get an orthosis

Footwear and orthoses can be obtained through the Orthotics Department in most hospitals and qualified orthotists are found there. Clear benefits to patients will occur if clinicians and orthotists together plan the indications and applications of orthoses for disabled people.

Table 12.1 Types of knee splint for particular injuries

Type of injury	Knee splint required
Mild collateral ligament injuries	A simple knee corset (e.g. neoprene) allows the patient to exercise quadriceps and hamstring muscles
More severe collateral ligament injuries	Full knee hinged corset for deformities of <20°. Little is of help for deformities of >20°
Cruciate ligament injuries	More complex stabilization from brace to prevent anteroposterior movement
Disrupted knees	Straight leg polythene jackets

Prostheses

Prostheses are devices which are often implanted and which aim to substitute the control of bodily functions, which have been impaired by disease, damage, or loss. The major prostheses encountered in rehabilitation refer to artificial limbs, joint replacement, and true implanted neurological prostheses. Artificial limbs will be discussed in further detail in Chapter 28.

Joint prostheses

Joint arthroplasty has revolutionized the management of chronic joint disease. Patients can now live their lives without pain and can virtually forget the severe disability to which they were formerly subjected by their arthritis. It is useful in both degenerative (osteoarthritis) and inflammatory joint disease and most experience has been gained from hip replacement. The use of superior techniques and materials has allowed greater survival of the prosthesis and one can now expect a hip arthroplasty to last for 10 to 15 years. Results tend to be better in osteoarthritis than in rheumatoid arthritis as bone quality and the integrity of the surrounding structures are more likely to be preserved. Reference to an orthopaedic or rheumatology textbook is recommended for further reading, but indications for surgery include nocturnal pain, loss of range of joint movement, such that function is impaired, progression of the underlying disease, and failure to respond adequately to medication and to physical treatment. Joint instability is not a contra-indication, but is likely to lead to a less favourable outcome if there is a significant deformity.

Various designs of the prosthesis are now available and surgery can replace either the whole joint or part of it. Many arthroplasty prostheses are now made of a mixture of metal and plastic to reduce load and give a longer life. Revision is possible if and when the prosthesis loosens, but requires great care in order to give the new artificial joint as much chance as possible of being as successful as the first. The major concern in arthroplasty operations is infection, and pain in a replaced joint should alert the physician to the presence of either infection or loosening of the prosthesis. Radiographs tend not to be of much help, but occasionally sclerosis around the root of the prosthesis can indicate loosening. The investigation of choice is an isotope bone scan using technetium-99, which shows the characteristic features of loosening. If infection is suspected, gamma scanning with gallium- or indium-labelled white cells can differentiate between acute and chronic inflammation. Gallium highlights lymphocytes, whereas indium targets polymorphonuclear white cells, and both are thus of great help. Infection requires prolonged antibiotic therapy for at least 6 to 12 weeks and may necessitate the removal of the prosthesis. The surgeon will have to be confident that infection has been irradicated before considering a new prosthesis.

Neuroprostheses

These are implantable devices which aim to improve functional independence and quality of life in people impaired by neurological disease, damage, or loss. They are not commonly used and therefore patients' relatives, carers, and rehabilitation professionals need to know what such devices can and cannot do. In addition, the latter need to have an understanding of the range of patients who may potentially benefit from their use. Neuroprostheses can be divided into three broad groups, which:

- Substitute for lost sensory functions (sensory prostheses).
- Substitute for lost motor functions (motor prostheses).
- Regulate deranged sensory or motor functions (neuromodulators).

Prostheses can result in either functional neurostimulation or functional substitution. The former differs in the time domain from all other forms of medical or surgical treatment and its impact on sensory or motor function can be controlled according to the functional requirements of the moment. At present, neurostimulation is fairly crude compared with that generated by the nervous system, but is improving all the time. A report on neuroprostheses and rehabilitation has recently been published by the British Society of Rehabilitation Medicine (*Neuroprostheses, Neuromodulators and Rehabilitation* (1997). Ed. D. Rushton. BSRM, London). Neuroprostheses may, for instance, be able to help people considerably but does not alter the underlying impairment. It reduces disability but is not a substitute for active rehabilitation. Rehabilitation is also about education, and the application of neuroprostheses must be accompanied by an educational process in their use and function. These devices are uncommon and therefore their prescription and fitting are limited to specialized centres. However, doctors referring into these centres should be certain that the present disabilities are unsatisfactorily managed and that the doctor, the patient, and the family agree that there is potential for further improvement with the use of an implant. Considerable motivation is required by some patients to gain anticipated benefits. Below is a list of some of the devices available implanted neuroprostheses:

- In use in most countries, many centres:
  - Cardiac pacemakers (for cardiac arrhythmias).
  - CSF shunts (for hydrocephalus).
- In use in several countries, specialized centres:
  - Spinal dorsal column stimulators (usually for pain).
  - Phrenic stimulators (for ventilation).
  - Cochlear stimulators (for profound deafness).
  - Baclofen pumps (for spasticity).
  - Bladder controllers (for continence and voiding).
- Establishing a clinical role, more than one centre:
  - Cerebellar stimulators (for spasticity, usually cerebral palsy)
  - Peroneal braces (for central foot-drop)
  - Activated gracilis slings (for anorectal incontinence).
  - Upper limb stimulators (for grasps in C5/6 quadriplegia).
- Investigational devices:
  - Lower limb stimulators (for paraplegic standing or walking).
  - Cerebellar stimulators (for epilepsy).
  - Visual cortex stimulators (for blindness).
  - Deep brain stimulators (for pain, tremor, or movement disorders).
  - Cavernosal drug pumps (for impotence).

Environmental control systems

One of the greatest benefits that modern technology has brought to the lives of disabled people is the ability to control their own lives at home. Opening the door to a caller, closing curtains, switching channels on the TV or radio seem such commonplace activities for able-bodied people, but an inability to do this can be very frustrating for disabled people. Furthermore, their carers are tied to the house and safety worries exist. Environmental control systems can change all this by providing a means for a person with a severe physical disability to control the access to his or her home, to summon emergency help, to operate everyday appliances such as the telephone, television etc., and to switch on and off electrical power for lighting and for other pieces of equipment. Increasing independence at home means that a disabled person can do much more of what he or she wishes in safety, thereby leaving carers free to get out of the house to gain much needed respite, as well as to do the shopping, etc.

Environmental control equipment has itself been subject to considerable technological advances, and visual display units are now commonplace. The use of radiowaves and infra-red has meant that direct electrical wiring linkages between the control box and the target appliances have now disappeared, making the home much safer for the disabled individual and for carers. No longer do people have to worry about tripping over wires. In addition, whereas separate switches were required for able-bodied members of the household, this is no longer the case and they can now operate the same appliances as the disabled person, which allows better integration for all concerned.

Organizational arrangements

Environmental control systems (ECS) are provided through regional centres in most parts of the country. A regional ECS coordinator is appointed to link in and liaise with local coordinators in each health district (usually occupational therapists working within a rehabilitation centre). The regional coordinator is also responsible for training, budget management, contract negotiation, supply and maintenance of equipment, and maintenance of the contract database. The local coordinator, on the other hand, has the task of patient follow-up, maintaining contract standards and local databases, and local liaison between users and professionals.

So how do disabled people get environmental control systems? Firstly, their attending professionals must have the training to have the systems in mind and know how they may be useful for a particular disabled individual. After the completed referral form is sent to the regional coordinator, a medical assessment is undertaken by a trained assessor, usually a consultant in rehabilitation medicine. The assessment includes the individual's other needs, as well as that of the environmental control system. The assessor reports back to the regional coordinator with detailed recommendations about the needs of the disabled individual and of potential solutions in the form of environmental control equipment. The client is then seen by the local coordinator, who is thereafter responsible for provision of equipment and coordination of delivery. Rehabilitation engineers assess the interface between the patient and the equipment within the home and the local coordinator will follow the individual up. Although environmental control systems are provided through the health budget, the wiring and any adaptations to the house require social services approval and funding and thus community occupational therapists also play an important role.

The equipment

Environmental controls usually comprise three different components:

- The selection unit, which acts as a nerve centre for the system.
- The input from the user to control the selection or new settings for various appliances.
- Commands to the controlled appliances.

Typical controlled appliances would be a door entry phone with an alarm or intercom system, light switches, telephone dialling systems, radio/TV/home entertainment control switches, and on and off facilities. Curtains and doors can also be opened and closed, but are usually extra items. The switches to control systems may be operated from a wheelchair or from a static surface, and various types are available. These include a hand-operated lever or joystick, a chin or headrest switch, suck and puff and pressure pad switches, as well as specialized inputs for picking up eye movements. The Steeper Fox and Possum Companion are some of the latest available models, but there are many older ones still in service which their users find more than satisfactory.

The assessment process

What should the assessment include? The medical history and its relevance to the assessment and the cause and progress of the disabling condition are of course important. The 24-h care profile and the hours in which a disabled person is to be left unattended must be documented. Many severely disabled people are not in fact left very much by their carers and this may be for two reasons. The first is that they do not actually wish to be left unattended and the second is that the carers are fearful of going out. Obviously, these aspects need to be tackled sensitively, but in these circumstances an environmental control may not be very useful and may end up as yet another piece of unused equipment in the house. In addition, opportunities for socializing are important and may require inclusion in the assessment. The health and needs of the carers require documentation, along with their burden of care and any physical or lifestyle restrictions they may have. The examination should not only include the individual's motor function, but their mental state, cognitive abilities, and their special senses (vision and hearing). It is obviously important that they can see the screen or listen to the bleep sounds. Surveying the environment will inform the assessor of other pieces of equipment currently in use. Unmet needs, both social and practical, also require documentation. Armed with this information, the assessment can then recommend a particular system and a trial may be necessary in order to identify whether or not the equipment is actually appropriate and of value.

Driving

Independent mobility has transformed the lives of some disabled people and new technologies have benefited people with even the most severe physical problems. Driving allows the disabled person to work, to maintain social contact, and to function independently in the community. It also encourages people to communicate and raises their self-esteem. Many cars, both big and small, come as standard, with automatic transmission, power-assisted steering, and electric windows, and are more reliable and easier to drive these days.

Disabled people require information about their suitability to drive and the following questions may be addressed.

• Their safety to drive.
• The most suitable type of car to acquire.
• Any aids and adaptations that are required.
• Sources of finance, purchase or hire of the vehicle.
• Insurance for driving and how to gain tax exemptions.
• How they can stow a wheelchair if one is used.
• How other people can be carried in the vehicle.
• How they can be assessed by an instructor with the necessary adaptations to a learner vehicle.
• Advice on alternative means of transportation if driving is not feasible.

The main medical barriers to driving are epilepsy, visual loss, cognitive deficits (in particular perceptual loss, memory loss, distraction and inattention, and intellectual loss), global dysphasia, severe mood changes and blackouts, dizziness etc. Loss of vision and perception mean that driving would be very difficult and it is incumbent that the rehabilitation team assesses this before raising the expectations of a disabled person to return to driving. Epilepsy is a proscribed condition for driving, for which the Department of Transport has guidelines. The ban on driving has been shortened in recent years, and 12 months of freedom from seizures while awake is the norm to allow return of a driving licence. This applies to a single fit as well as to post-traumatic epilepsy. Nocturnal epilepsy, when seizures occur during sleep, must not have been present for 3 years.

Vehicle modifications

Virtually anything it seems nowadays can be done to a vehicle to make it suitable for a disabled person to drive. However, transportation is not only about a disabled person getting behind the steering wheel. Access is also an issue. Vehicles can be adapted to allow transfer from a wheelchair to a car seat, or by build modification to allow the disabled person to travel in his or her own wheelchair in the vehicle. A whole host of seat cushions, steering aids, and hand-operated controls (brakes, accelerators, etc.) can be fitted in or after manufacture so that specific adaptations do not necessarily need to be made. Certain items are now indispensable, such as a car telephone, in order to summon help quickly, if required.

Many rehabilitation centres are able to assess people on their own premises, but the Forum of UK Mobility Centres see large numbers of people. Interestingly, many otherwise able-bodied people also undertake a disabled driving assessment on their 70th birthday in order to give them the confidence to continue driving beyond that age.

Chapter 13

Behavioural disorders

Background

Problems with behaviour are regrettably quite common in rehabilitation units, particularly those dealing with people with traumatic brain injury. The period of confusion during post-traumatic amnesia can often lead to inappropriate behaviour. Fortunately in most people behavioural problems are relatively mild and short-lived. It is only a minority who develop longer-term persistent and seriously disruptive behaviour. This group will often need specialist assistance from a neurobehavioural unit. However, the majority can, and should, be adequately managed in a rehabilitation unit. Almost all units, and particularly those catering for people with traumatic brain injury, should have access to a clinical neuropsychologist who is likely to be the leading figure in assessment and management of people with behavioural disorders.

Behavioural problems can follow any brain injury but are most common following traumatic brain injury. They are also particularly common after anoxic brain injury and less so after stroke or multiple sclerosis. It is also worth remembering that people with pre-existing behavioural problems secondary to mental illness or learning disabilities can also suffer traumatic brain injury and exhibit a worsening (or sometimes an improvement) of their previous difficulties.

Behavioural problems can be grouped into two broad categories: inappropriate excessive behaviour and inappropriate lack of behaviour. The former, which is the commoner form after traumatic brain injury, can present with a variety of difficulties:

- verbal aggression
- physical aggression
- shouting at staff members or other clients
- aggressive refusal to cooperate with the rehabilitation programme
- inappropriate sexual behaviour
- impulsivity
- extreme egocentrism.

The most dramatic end of the behavioural spectrum is termed 'episodic dyscontrol syndrome'. In this syndrome the individual can have sudden aggressively violent outbursts with little or no warning.

At the other end of the spectrum inappropriate lack of behaviour can include:

- apathy
- lack of initiation
- requirement for prompting and cajoling to undertake simple daily living tasks.

In these circumstances individuals are often labelled as lacking in motivation. Such a label should be avoided. The implication of lack of motivation or laziness is that it is the fault of the individual and therefore there is little that can be done to correct the problem. Such a label can produce a nihilistic approach to therapy which is in no-one's interest.

Learning theory

Behavioural management techniques are normally based on various classical learning theories. Thus a brief overview of learning theory is desirable. This is a complex and specialist subject and this brief description will have to be simplistic. There are three broad areas of learning theory:

- classical conditioning
- operant conditioning
- observational or vicarious conditioning.

Classical conditioning

This is classical Pavlovian theory and explains behaviour in terms of learning that two stimuli tend to go together. In his classic experiments Pavlov showed that a dog salivated on presentation of a stimulus such as a bell or light if, on previous occasions, this stimulus had been associated with the presentation of food. The bell or light is known as the *conditional stimulus* and the salivation as the *conditional response*. This association can be broken if one stimulus becomes unassociated with the other—known as extinction. Sometimes the association can also generalize with similar conditional stimuli, such as a different light or a different sound.

Operant conditioning

Operant or instrumental conditioning occurs when individuals correctly learn the association between some action of their own and an environmental consequence. This can include the delivery of food or giving praise. Procedures adapted from operant conditioning studies form the majority of behavioural modification techniques.

Classical and operant conditioning are both forms of associative learning. In other words the individual learns a linkage between one experience and another. There is now good evidence, particularly from animal studies, that associative learning abilities are retained even in the presence of severe brain damage. Associative learning has even been demonstrated when people are still in coma. This is why associative learning techniques are the most successful in those with brain damage.

Observational or vicarious conditioning

This is learning that occurs through observation. A child, for example, can learn to be fearful of spiders if the parent is seen to be frightened. It is likely that such learning requires relatively intact cognitive processes. Cognitive approaches to retraining are usually more relevant when cognitive impairments are specific rather than more global.

Approaches to the management of behavioural problems: definition of the problem

There are two questions that need to be answered here:
- What is the problem?
- Who has the problem?

What is the problem?

The answers must be tightly defined. It is insufficient to say that X is aggressive. X may only be aggressive in particular circumstances or with particular people or doing particular things.

Who has the problem?

Sometimes the behavioural problem in the individual is relatively mild but has been overemphasized or exaggerated by carers, family or staff. Sometimes staff could require the individual to be at a particular place at a particular time—say for medication or at mealtimes. If the individual is not in the right place at the right time then they may be labelled as having behavioural disorders whereas in fact they may not be hungry or not agree with the necessity of being at a particular place.

Once it is agreed by all concerned that there is a problem with a particular behaviour then it needs further analysis.

Approaches to the management of behavioural problems: study and analyse the problem

A useful approach is ABC—Antecedent, Behaviour, Consequence. In order to further analyse the problem individuals will need to be carefully observed. If resources permit then this is best done by a dedicated member of staff over a prolonged period of time. It is usually difficult, if not impossible, for an individual's behaviour to be properly studied and analysed on a busy rehabilitation ward without some dedicated staff time.

The *antecedent* behaviour determines what pre-dates or seems to trigger the inappropriate behaviour. Different questions to ask include:

- In what circumstances does it occur?
- What appears to trigger it?
- What appears not to trigger it?
- Is it situation specific?
- Is it environment specific?
- Is it person specific?
- Is there no pattern at all?

Next, the *behaviour* itself needs close analysis:

- What are the characteristics of the behaviour?
- What form does it take?
- How long does it last?
- To whom is it directed?
- To what is it directed?
- How often does it occur?

Next, *consequence* (what are the consequences of the behaviour?):

- Is there an observed benefit?
- Does it lead to reward or another form of positive reinforcement?
- Does the individual calm down quickly or slowly?

After such a period of close observation a pattern usually emerges—it is unusual for behavioural disturbance not to be triggered by anything and to have no pattern at all.

Approaches to the management of behavioural problems: formulate the treatment plan (i)

After definition and study of the problem it is usually possible to define a specific behaviour that is to be targeted. It is usually best to work on one or a very few behaviours at any one time. As with all rehabilitation processes a measuring instrument needs to be devised in order to monitor the defined goal. Intangible outcomes, such as X is less aggressive, are not adequate. Specific measures are required, such as how many times X is aggressive over a given period of time or at a particular time of the day. Specific goals will often require continued close observation, and this in turn often still requires a dedicated and trained member of staff to undertake observation.

Specific treatment methodologies: increasing desirable behaviours

Desirable behaviours can be increased in a number of different ways. The commonest method is by *positive reinforcement*. A positive reinforcement is something which is delivered immediately following the occurrence of a positive behaviour which will increase the probability of that behaviour being repeated. Such reinforcement should be as close to the behaviour as possible. The reinforcement can be tangible, such as food and drink, less tangible, such as praise, or be a conditionary reinforcer where the person must learn the relative value of the reinforcement by receiving, for example, tokens. The tokens can then be exchanged for later secondary reinforcers, such as coffee or snacks.

The reinforcement should be given immediately after the behaviour occurs and in a consistent and clear manner. All members of the rehabilitation unit must know the behavioural approaches being adopted so that every time a particular behaviour occurs it can be appropriately reinforced by the same means.

There are a number of other related techniques:

- *Shaping*. Shaping involves reinforcement of the small steps towards an eventual desired behaviour. If, for example, someone refuses to dress in the mornings then they could be initially rewarded for just looking at their clothes, then perhaps touching the clothes or putting them in an appropriate place and then rewarded step by step over a period of time for each item of clothing that is correctly put on. Eventually the small reinforcers are withdrawn and larger steps, such as dressing the top half of the body without prompts, are reinforced until finally positive reinforcement is only given after completion of the entire task.
- *Fading* can occur if prompting is required and after some time that level of prompt is withdrawn.
- *Modelling* is imitation of the desired behaviour by a member of staff and such imitation is slowly withdrawn. This observational conditioning will often require a higher degree of cognitive function than the more simple associative learning techniques.

- *Environmental restructuring* this is sometimes needed in order to reduce the chances that a situation occurs in which the behaviour can be triggered. If, for example, someone easily gets angry if they cannot coordinate their cutlery and plate then use of non-slip mats, plate guards and adapted cutlery could make eating easier and reduce inappropriate behaviours.

Approaches to the management of behavioural problems: formulate the treatment plan (ii)

Specific treatment methodologies: decreasing undesirable behaviours

There are two basic methods to decrease undesirable behaviours:

- *Punishment* involves the presentation of an aversive stimulus or removal of a positive stimulus immediately following the inappropriate behaviour.
- *Extinction* occurs when the reinforcer is no longer delivered to a previously reinforced response.

There are various forms of punishment:

- *Time out on the spot* (TOOTS): this involves denying attention to behaviours, such as screaming or complaining, by either, for example, continuing with a conversation as if oblivious to the behaviour or simply by walking away.
- *Situational time out*: this involves removal of the person either from the activity to another part of the room or to a separate room, without providing verbal reinforcement.
- *Seclusion time out* is where the individual is placed in a bare room for periods of about 5 min—there are now doubts about whether this can be ethically justified.
- *Response cost*: if a token economy is being used to reward someone after positive behaviour then the same tokens can be removed after inappropriate behaviour.

Overall these techniques do require a considerable amount of skill, planning, and staff time. The programme can take several weeks to have an effect and sometimes it can be very difficult to generalize behavioural improvements into a broader setting. Some authorities say that such behavioural management programmes cannot really be applied in a general rehabilitation or hospital environment. However, in non-specialist units small-scale specific behavioural alterations can be made, although staff time and resources can be a problem.

Drug therapy

Behavioural management programmes should not rely on the use of sedative, anxiolytic, or psychotropic medication. Indeed such drugs can often worsen behaviour. Occasionally the use of such a drug on a general medical ward where there is real risk to other staff or patients can be justified but, in general, drugs should be avoided in the management of any behavioural disorder. There are some exceptions. In the more severe explosive forms of behaviour—the episodic dyscontrol syndrome—then anti-convulsants can be helpful, including carbamazepine and gabapentin.

Some would use the serotoninergic anti-depressant, trazodone, whilst others would advocate the use of lithium or beta blockade with metoprolol. If severe agitation requires treatment then buspirone is useful. Individuals with inappropriate lack of behaviour can sometimes respond to central stimulants such as dexamphetamine or methylphenidate, but such medication should be used with caution.

Approaches to the management of behavioural problems: evaluation

After an appropriate period of intervention the behavioural strategy will need evaluation and perhaps the strategy itself or the goals will need readjustment. Behavioural management is a dynamic phenomenon and specific goals and targets will need constant review. However, unlike some aspects of physical rehabilitation behavioural rehabilitation can take many months. Severe behavioural problems can take a year or more to change and are sometimes very resistant to generalization into other settings. Fortunately many behaviours arising in the recovery phase of traumatic brain injury, particularly around the period of emergence from post-traumatic amnesia, are short-lived and generally responsive to behavioural manipulation.

Overall, behavioural disorders are quite common following brain injury and can be a significant source of disruption to the rehabilitation programme. However, in most people such behaviours are short-lived and can be relatively easily managed by a simple behavioural management approach. However, even simple behaviours can be time-consuming for staff and must be delivered in a consistent fashion by the whole unit as well as by carers and family. Despite the problems, behavioural intervention can produce gratifying improvements for many people and enable them to lead a more independent life where otherwise some form of restrictive environment may have been necessary.

Psychiatric problems and rehabilitation

Background

People with physical disabilities are not immune to psychiatric problems and people with psychiatric problems are not immune to acquiring physical disability as a result of trauma or disease. People with some specific psychiatric problems such as personality disorders, substance abuse, and alcoholism are particularly prone to acquiring physical disability, secondary to risk-taking or risk-attracting behaviour. In addition, brain injury itself can be associated with specific psychiatric problems. There is still much debate about whether such difficulties as depression, anxiety, or more profound problems such as psychosis are secondary to intrinsic brain damage or simply a secondary result of a reaction to such damage. In the end the causation is of little consequence as individuals will still need appropriate psychiatric assistance. There is no evidence that a person, for example, with depression in the context of physical disability is any more or less likely to respond to appropriate treatment than someone with an endogenous or reactive depression.

Rehabilitation units should obviously have access to a skilled multidisciplinary psychiatric team, particularly for people with more profound or chronic psychiatric problems. The following sections do not attempt to be a substitute for a psychiatric textbook but the management of the commonest psychiatric problems should certainly be part of the armamentarium of the rehabilitation team. Many rehabilitation units use some form of screening questionnaire to detect psychiatric problems, particularly depression and anxiety. Regrettably many self-report mood scales include a variety of somatic symptoms, which in themselves can be part of the associated physical disability. Such symptoms might include insomnia, weight loss, anorexia, early morning waking, and loss of libido. Thus, it may be best to use mood scales that exclude such somatic symptoms. Two scales worth noting are:

- The Hospital Anxiety and Depression Scale.[1]
- The Wimbledon Self Report Scale.[2]

Both these scales exclude somatic items and are valid and reliable as screening measures for anxiety and depression. The *General Health Questionnaire* (GHQ 28) is also well developed as a screening measure for depression and anxiety but does include somatic and social dimensions.[3]

These scales should not be used as the only measures of assessment, but are useful screening tools; appropriate cut off points could be used for further referral to an appropriate psychiatric or psychological assessment.

The commonest psychiatric problems encountered in rehabilitation units include depression, anxiety, post-traumatic stress disorder, and emotional lability.

Depression

Depressive illness is remarkably common after acquired physical disability. It occurs in around 50% of people following stroke and severe head injury. It is even commoner at some point during progressive neurological disability, such as multiple sclerosis and motor neuron disease. People with congenital disabilities or childhood-acquired disabilities also have periods when they are particularly prone to depression. This is often true at times of life change, such as around puberty or when striving to be independent and leaving the parental home.

There is a continuum of depressive illness, from feeling temporarily low to sustained major depression with risk of suicide. The current accepted classification is usually based on the American Psychiatric Association criteria published as a Diagnostic and Statistical Manual for Psychiatric Disorders (DSM IV). However, such a formal diagnosis is probably not necessary in the setting of rehabilitation unit.

Depression is usually characterised by:
• Sustained unpleasant mood either described directly as depression or as sadness, unhappiness, or the inability to feel pleasure (anhedonia).

There are behavioural accompaniments, such as:
• social withdrawal,
• physical slowing,
• crying,
cognitive accompaniments:
• ideas of hopelessness, worthlessness and guilt,
physiological or biological accompaniments:
• anorexia,
• weight loss,
• insomnia,
• early morning waking,
• loss of libido.

Treatment of depression

There are various labels for the different forms of depression including *adjustment disorder* (temporarily linked to a stressor; tends to resolve over less than 6 months) or *major depression* (more severe and more persistent). However, the label is less important than the diagnosis and determination of whether it is actually contributing to an impairment of function. If depression is adversely affecting function in any way then treatment should be initiated. There are two broad approaches:

- psychological strategies
- psychotropic medication.

Psychological strategies

Psychological strategies depend primarily on an understanding and sympathetic relationship between the counsellor, psychologist or psychotherapist, and the person with depression. The following points are key to appropriate management:

- Information about and explanation of the nature of the depression.
- Detailed exploration of ideas and knowledge about the person's illness and their views on prognosis.
- A broad-ranging discussion on the overall impact of the physical illness and depressive illness on the family, social, and work relationships.
- Discussion to bring out potential stressors and triggers to day-to-day variations in mood.
- Development of coping strategies.

There are various specific counselling or psychotherapeutic approaches that have been used and published and it is not appropriate or possible in this section to go through these strategies. However, the following may be used:

- Cognitive behavioural therapy.
- Client-centred approach of Karl Rogers.
- Rational emotive therapy.
- Gestalt therapy.

There are other approaches that may

- improve motivation,
- increase treatment adherence, and
- overcome apathy and inertia.

It is important to note that many anti-depressive cognitive strategies do require a reasonably intact cortex and may be inappropriate for those with more severe forms of brain damage. In such people some would advocate the use of medication.

Medication

Medication does have an important place in the management of acute affective disorders and in the prevention of recurrent problems. The following are frequently used:

- Lithium for bipolar disorders.
- Older tricyclic anti-depressants (amitriptyline, dothiepin, clomipramine, and imipramine): these are useful anti-depressants but usage is often limited by troublesome anti-cholinergic side-effects (urinary retention

and constipation and dry mouth are of particular relevance in the physically disabled population) and sedative properties.
• Newer tetracyclic anti-depressants and 5HT uptake inhibitors (such as fluoxetine and fluvoxamine).
• Specialist use of other anti-depressant agents, such as monoamine-oxidase inhibitors or, for severe mood swings, anti-convulsants, such as carbamazepine.
• ECT in the most severe cases.

The latter categories should probably only be used by a formal psychiatric team.

Anti-depressant medication should be used for several months and most authorities would recommend continuation of medication for at least 6 months and probably longer in more severe cases.

Anxiety

Anxiety, like depression, is a common companion to physical disability. Anxiety also has physiological, behavioural, and cognitive accompaniments. Symptoms can include:

- Feeling of fearful anticipation.
- Irritability.
- Restlessness.
- Worry.
- Poor concentration.
- Feeling of tightness in the chest or difficulty breathing.
- Cardiovascular symptoms, such as palpitations.
- Gastrointestinal symptoms, such as dry mouth, difficulty swallowing, loose bowel motions.
- Musculoskeletal problems, such as ache and tension in the scalp, neck, or shoulders.
- Sleep problems, such as difficulty getting to sleep and restless sleep.
- Appetite disturbance.
- Central nervous system problems, such as blurring of vision, paraesthesia, and dizziness.
- Avoidance of anxiety-provoking situation, such as agoraphobia.
- Avoidance of physical activity or even avoidance of human company.

The latter problems, in a rehabilitation setting, can be interpreted as anti-social behaviour or lack of initiative and drive which are simply secondary to the brain injury, whereas treatment of the anxiety state may produce benefit.

Treatment

Psychological problems and/or medication can be used and include:

- Specific anxiety management training programmes, including relaxation techniques and distraction techniques.
- Specific counselling techniques as listed in the section on depression above.
- Anxiolytic medication—this should be avoided if possible but benzodiazepines are relatively safe and effective anxiolytics. Treatment should, if at all possible, be short term. Withdrawal can be difficult with a risk of rebound anxiety.
- Anti-depressants will often have anti-anxiety effect and can be used even in the absence of depression.

It is very important to stress that anxiety can be caused or certainly worsened by insufficient information and explanation about current or potential new symptoms or about the natural history or prognosis of the disorder. Effective and sympathetic communication is probably the best anxiolytic and thus appropriate prevention and management is the responsibility of the whole rehabilitation team.

Post-traumatic stress disorder

Post-traumatic stress disorder can occur after anyone has been exposed to a traumatic event. The seriousness of the event is not necessarily a good guide to the severity of the symptoms as individuals will respond differently to the same stressors. Paradoxically the most severe brain injuries are usually associated with a period of post-traumatic amnesia and inability to recall the traumatic event and some authorities have said that post-traumatic stress disorder cannot, by definition, exist in such people. This is probably not true as individuals can develop symptoms after being told the details of the accident or trauma. There are specific diagnostic criteria published by the American Psychiatric Association (DSM IV). Basically the diagnosis rests on:

- Persistent re-experience of the event.
- Recurrent or intrusive distressing recollections.
- Recurrent or intrusive distressing nightmares related to the event.
- Avoidance of the scene of the trauma.
- Intense distress secondary to various triggers that symbolize or resemble part of the event.

The latter will result in efforts to avoid thoughts or feelings about the trauma and feelings of detachment or estrangement from others.

There are often persistent symptoms of:

- Increased arousal.
- Difficulty falling asleep.
- Irritability.
- Problems with concentration.
- Exaggerated startle response.

In many people these symptoms are relatively minor and short-lived. However, in others the symptoms can be persistent and long term and have a major effect on lifestyle and quality of life.

In such people specific psychological referral should be made as a number of treatment strategies have been shown to be beneficial. Cognitive behavioural therapy, for example, is useful as are various forms of group therapy, and if the problem has a bearing on the whole family then couple therapy or family therapy can be helpful.

Medication should be avoided, but depression and anxiety symptoms, which may need medication, can co-exist.

Emotionalism

A number of disorders affecting the brain can lead to disturbance of emotionality—disturbance of the normal control or expression of emotion. There are two syndromes:
- pathological crying and laughing
- emotional lability.

Pathological crying and laughing

This is provoked by non-emotional stimuli. There is no affect that accompanies the pathological laughing and crying. The emotional expression cannot be controlled and the emotional behaviour is stereotyped.

Emotional lability

This is produced by emotionally appropriate stimuli and often will look like normal crying or laughing but the trigger for such lability appears to be set at a different level from the 'normal' population. However, the distinction between these two syndromes is blurred and many would now prefer the term emotionalism for both phenomena.

The problem is probably a direct manifestation of brain pathology rather than indicating any underlying emotional disturbance. Obviously a diagnosis of co-existent depression, anxiety, or post-traumatic stress disorder can be very difficult in such circumstances. However, emotionalism does seem to respond quite well to small doses of anti-depressant medication. The response can be dramatic to doses that would not normally be expected to have an anti-depressive effect. Sometimes modest doses of anti-convulsant medication, particularly carbamazepine, can also be helpful.

References

1 Zigmond, A. and Snaith, P. (1983). Hospital Anxiety and Depression Scale. *Acta Psychiatrica Scandinvacia* **67**: 361–70.

2 Coughlan, A. and Storey, P. (1988). The Wimbledon Self Report Scale: emotional mood appraisal. *Clinical Rehabilitation* **2**: 207–13.

3 Goldberg, D.P. and Hillier, V.F. (1979). A scaled version of the General Health Questionnaire. *Psychological Medicine* **9**: 139–45.

Chapter 15

Cognitive and intellectual function

Background and terminology

Cognition is the term that refers to all the processes involved in perceiving, learning, remembering, and thinking. Thus, cognitive problems are very common in any process that affects brain function. The key to helping people with cognitive problems is accurate assessment of the nature of the problem. This should be followed by clear-cut information and advice about the nature of the problem—both to the affected person and the family. Until recent years neurologists and neuropsychologists had to stop at this point as there was little functional assistance that could be offered. This is now less true, and there are a number of useful strategies designed to improve various cognitive problems or at least to help the individual cope with them better. Cognitive rehabilitation is a relatively new and largely untested field but rapid progress is being made.

The terminology used in cognitive assessment can be confusing and the following two sections offer a very simple guide to cognitive terminology.

Perceptual problems

Perception is the cognitive process that enables us to make sense of our environment. This can be through any of the senses but the most important are:

- *Sight*—visual perception.
- *Hearing*—auditory perception.
- *Touch*—tactile perception.

Perceptual deficits of taste and smell do exist but in humans are of less functional significance. Perception can be affected in a number of ways.

Agnosia

Agnosia is the inability to perceive that cannot be explained by a primary sensory disorder or a deficit of naming or severe general intellectual impairment. Each of the senses has a specific agnosia. Visual agnosia is the most important.

Thus, *visual agnosia* is the inability to recognize objects which cannot be explained on the basis of a primary sight disorder or on the basis of a language problem or general intellectual loss. There are more precise visual agnostic syndromes including:

- *Colour agnosia*—loss of the ability to recognize colours.
- *Prosopagnosia*—loss of the ability to recognize familiar faces.
- *Simultanagnosia*—loss of the ability to perceive all the elements of a scene simultaneously and interpret that scene, i.e. recognition of parts of the scene but not the whole.

The other senses also have their own forms of agnosia, such as tactile agnosia and auditory agnosia.

Neglect

Neglect is the failure to attend to one side of a space or one side of self by the relevant sense. Individuals with *visual neglect*, for example, will commonly bump into things on the affected side or fail to see food on one side of the plate thinking they have finished the meal when in fact it has only been half eaten. This is commonly, but not always, a right-hemisphere problem and is particularly common after stroke.

Apraxias

These are perceptual problems in which a person without general intellectual decline and without weakness, ataxia, motor, or sensory deficit is unable to execute previously learnt skills or gestures. The apraxias can be subdivided into:

- *Ideational apraxia*—where there is a complete failure to conceive or formulate an action either spontaneously and/or to a command.
- *Ideomotor apraxia*—where the individual knows and remembers the plan of action but simply cannot carry it out.

There can be quite specific forms of apraxia including:

- *Constructional apraxia*—refers to problems in putting things together in two or three dimensions, such as jigsaw puzzles.

- *Dressing apraxia*—the inability to dress properly and remember the right clothing in the right sequence. This is common after stroke and can lead to people being completely unable to dress or, in less serious cases, simply trying to put their trousers on the wrong way around or putting underpants on after the trousers.

Language and communication problems

These are discussed elsewhere but language problems are a common accompaniment to other cognitive difficulties.

Dysphasia

Dysphasia is a generic term for the understanding of language. It is usually divided into non-fluent and fluent aphasias:

- Non-fluent aphasia usually corresponds to damage to the anterior part of the brain. As a generalization people with such aphasias have great difficulty in expressing themselves with the correct words in the right sequence. Part of the non-fluent aphasic syndrome used to be known as Broca's aphasia. There are now recognized to be three basic non-fluent aphasias—*Broca's aphasia*, *transcortical motor aphasia*, and *global aphasia*. The distinction between these aphasias is outside the scope of this volume.

- Fluent aphasias tend to result from damage to the posterior part of the brain and tend to lead to problems of understanding or comprehension. These used to be called receptive dysphasias and a well-known variety is Wernicke's aphasia. Once again there are now recognized to be three forms of fluent aphasia—*Wernicke's aphasia*, *transcortical sensory aphasia*, and *conduction aphasia*.

The subtleties of the classification are certainly important in making a formal functional assessment and are becoming important in terms of remediation of various communication problems. These difficulties are in the realm of the specialist speech and language therapist.

The various dysphasias do need to be distinguished from *dysarthria*, which is a problem of speech production usually due to brainstem or local mouth or pharyngeal pathology. Classically the individual has a slurring of speech, and once again there are various defined subtypes.

There is other language terminology:

- *Anomia*—specific naming ability causing problems naming particular objects.
- *Paraphasia*—production of an unintended or nonsense word (neologism).
- *Agrammaticism*—difficulty with grammar or structure of language.
- Various disorders causing problems with repetition.
- Problems repeating phrases.
- Often people with problems of language processing have related difficulties with reading (*dyslexia*), writing (*dysgraphia*), and calculating (*dyscalculia*).

Memory problems

Memory problems are probably the commonest cognitive problem following brain injury and the one that has the most profound impact on daily function. There has recently been much progress in the understanding of memory and some progress (see later) in rehabilitation of memory difficulties. There are a number of dimensions of memory.

Different time spans

- *Immediate or working memory*. This is memory just for the previous few seconds, such as is required to hold a telephone number in the head whilst dialling. There are different forms of working memory according to the different senses used—*phrenological system* for auditory information, *visuo-spatial system* for visual information as well as a *controlling central executive system*.
- *Long-term memory*:
  - *Delayed*—memory for events that happened in the previous few minutes.
  - *Recent*—memory for events that happened in the previous days or weeks.
  - *Remote*—memory for events that happened several weeks to several years previously.
- *Prospective memory*. Memory for things that need to be done in the future.

Different types of information

- *Semantic memory*—memory for factual knowledge.
- *Episodic memory*—memory for events and autobiographical material.
- *Procedural memory*—memory for skills and practical procedures; this is often preserved in brain injury when episodic and semantic memory is not.

Memory in different forms

- *Verbal memory*—memory for information in the form of words, both written and spoken.
- *Visual memory*—memory for things that have to be remembered in visual format.

Stages of remembering

All these different forms of memory need to go through different stages of encoding, storage, and later retrieval. Problems can arise at any of these stages for any of the different memories and thus one can see the complexity of trying to unravel the different forms of memory disorder.

Perhaps an example is useful. Remembering how to drive a car is a skill that will require procedural memory. The fact that a car is used to drive one to work is semantic memory and the fact that the car was actually used to drive to work that morning needs episodic memory. Memory that the car is made of metal and the tyres of rubber is semantic memory. There may be other memories about different cars that one has purchased in the past or particularly pleasant or unpleasant memories about particular cars.

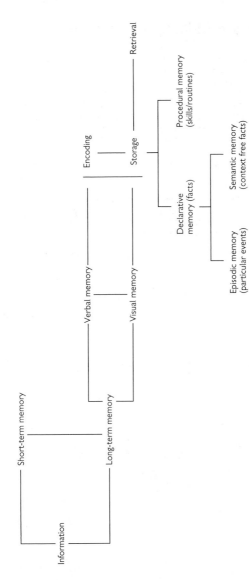

Fig. 15.1 Long- and short-term memory.

Memory problems (*continued*)

A few other memory terms need to be described:

- *Retrograde amnesia* is usually associated with cerebral injury and applies to loss of memory prior to the injury, which is usually a very short period of time and normally only a few minutes.
- *Anterograde amnesia* applies to on-going memory disturbance after a particular trauma. The commonest form is *post-traumatic amnesia* (PTA), which describes the period of time after a cerebral insult before continuous day-to-day memory returns. The length of PTA is a good determinant of the severity of the injury and the prognosis for later recovery.

Memory is undoubtedly complicated and Fig. 15.1 illustrates a simple schematic summarizing, probably in an over-simplistic form, the different forms of memory.

Psychologists now have a number of standardized tests for assessment of the different forms of memory and a clinical neuropsychologist should be involved in the assessment and treatment of anyone with a memory problem, or indeed other cognitive problems.

Attention deficits and other problems of higher executive function

Attention is the ability to remain aware of one's surroundings. It is also the ability to selectively attend to important signals. One may be listening, for example, to music and can divert attention if someone starts a conversation even though the music is still playing. Problems with attention can easily result in difficulties with daily living. People with brain injuries have problems with *selective attention* and find it difficult to exclude less important inputs—the so-called cocktail party syndrome. At a party, for example, they may not be able to selectively attend to the person with whom they are talking if there are other background conversations or music. They may also have problems *alternating attention* from one task to another, such as when driving a car. They may have problems with *dividing attention* in order to respond simultaneously to two or more things at once, such as carrying on a conversation whilst driving.

There is also a cluster of symptoms that people classically show following damage to the frontal lobe brain structures. People with such damage often experience a large range of difficulties in everyday life. These symptoms used to be called the 'frontal lobe syndrome'. However, this label is rather unsatisfactory and implies a clear-cut syndrome. It is more helpful to categorize the particular problems in an individual person and the whole collection of symptoms is now known as the 'dysexecutive syndrome'. There are a number of characteristics which can be listed:

- Problems with abstract thinking.
- Impulsivity.
- Confabulation.
- Problems with planning.
- Euphoria.
- Temporal sequencing problems.
- Lack of insight and social awareness.
- Apathy and lack of drive.
- Disinhibition.
- Disturbed impulse control.
- Shallow affective responses.
- Aggression.
- Lack of concern.
- Perseveration.
- Restlessness.
- Inability to inhibit responses.
- Distractibility.
- Loss of decision-making ability.
- Lack of concern for social rules.

A look down this list will indicate the very wide variety of problems that can occur in the dysexecutive syndrome and the difficulties that can result in terms of everyday life and social functioning.

Cognitive rehabilitation

Is it possible to restore cognitive function? This has been a controversial question for a number of years and there is still limited evidence to make a definitive answer. Placebo-controlled, double-blind studies are very difficult, and some would say impossible, in this field and scientific progress has usually relied on single-case methodology. There is now some evidence that a number of cognitive problems are amenable to a rehabilitation strategy, including:

- Attention deficits.
- Unilateral neglect.
- Some deficits in communication, including dyslexia.
- Some aspects of memory dysfunction.

In broad terms functional benefit can derive from a broad cognitive approach that adopts two strategies:

- Bypass the problem or find another way to achieve the same goal.
- Use residual skills more effectively.

Finding a way around the problem

A number of strategies can be designed according to the individual problems. People can be provided with assistive equipment. Individuals with memory problems, for example, can be taught to use external memory aids, such as diaries, lists, alarm clocks, timers, and tape recorders. However, this is not always successful as people need some residual memory in order to remember what they are being reminded about! There are commercial systems that are radio-controlled and a central switchboard will transmit a message into a small communicator reminding the person what needs doing at that particular moment.

Another strategy is to rearrange the immediate environment in order to reduce cognitive input. Sometimes this will involve a rigid organization of daily life so that limited planning and organizational skills are required. A very structured day, with diaries and prompts from another party, can often assist someone with aspects of the dysexecutive syndrome. Organization of physical space, such as labelling draws, doors and kitchen utensils can be helpful. Sometimes simple measures can help such as supplying simple clothing with labels and Velcro fastening for people with dressing apraxia. There are a whole variety of strategies that first need an accurate neuropsychological assessment and then application of a common-sense way to get around the problem.

Using residual skills more effectively

There are a number of techniques in this area that have mainly been developed in the field of memory. Mnemonic strategies have been used including *imagery*, where information is remembered by an association with a particular image. An example is the *PQRST* mnemonic. In this technique individuals are taught to Preview information, set Questions to themselves on the information, Read information over, State the information again, and Test the results. It is hoped by this method that the information is more deeply encoded. There are many other techniques that can use acronyms, rhymes, and systematic cueing, where a well-known series, such as the alphabet, is scanned through to cue an appropriate memory. This, and many other techniques, are designed to use residual skills more efficiently and now have been shown to produce real functional benefit and lessen disability in many people. In an individual case a number of different strategies can be used. It is vital that the main carers and family are involved in the regular and routine implementation of an appropriate strategy.

Participation issues in rehabilitation

Introduction

Participation issues are concerned with the factors that affect the lives of people with disabilities. Although often outside the control of health professionals, as they are based on societal attitudes and governmental legislative policy, the rehabilitation team needs to develop links with professionals in employment, social services, and housing departments. This chapter has a UK orientation, but the same principles apply in other countries.

Finance and benefits

Typical problems faced are:

- *Low income.* Low income is one of the greatest barriers to participation for disabled people. Although paid employment is a valid goal for many younger people, work for many middle-aged and older people will not be realistic because of their functional restriction or because of societal barriers. Many disabled people have a low income from being unemployed, having to work part-time, or working in menial or low-paid jobs.
- *Increased expenditure*: equipment, increased clothing needs and heating costs, contributions to housing adaptations, travel, etc.

The benefits structure is very complicated and many people do not know what they are entitled to. Help is at hand in most towns and cities through Citizens' Advice Bureaux and information desks of disabled peoples' organizations, such as DIAL. Rehabilitation teams should have a working knowledge of people's rights on welfare and should know the appropriate information sources in their community. Table 16.1 gives a summary of some of the benefits.

Table 16.1 Summary of UK benefits

Situation	Benefit available
Incapable of work: previously employed	Statutory Sick Pay for 28 weeks. Incapacity Benefit >28 weeks
Eligible for Incapacity Benefit (IB): Short-term sick for 28–52 weeks Long-term sick for >52 weeks ± receiving high rate of Disability Living Allowance care component IB started before age of 45 years	Short-term IB Long-term IB Incapacity Age Addition
Incapable of work: ≥16 h work/week for ≥4 weeks, ≥16 years of age with disability or aged ≥25 years and usually working for ≥30h/week	Disabled Person's Working Tax Credit
Incapable of work: ≥16 h work/week for ≥4 weeks, ≥16 years of age with disability or aged ≥25 years and usually working for ≥30hrs/week and looking after child dependants	Child Tax Credit
<60 years. Incapable of work and insufficient to live on—means tested, minimum income guaranteed	Income Support
Unemployed	Income Support/Jobseeker's Allowance
Incapable of full-time work, but working <16h per week	Jobseeker's Allowance
Incapable of work from industrial injury or work-related illness	Industrial Injuries Disablement Benefit
War disablement	War Disablement Pension / War Widows' Pension
Disabled person aged <65 years requiring help with Personal care Mobility	Disability Living Allowance Care component—low, middle, and high rates Mobility component—low and high rates 'Motability' loan for vehicular transport Blue Badge parking from local authority Road tax exemption
Disabled person aged ≥65 years requiring help with personal care	Attendance Allowance
Injury due to violent crime	Criminal Injuries Compensation
Vaccine damage	Vaccine damage payment
Help with living at home and requiring home improvements while on income support	Housing Benefit, Council Tax Benefit
Other	Bus/rail pass for all aged ≥60 years

Education and further education

Children with disabilities have to remain in education until the age of 16 years, but further education facilities are available to the age of 19 years. The policy has been for many years to educate disabled children as far as possible in mainstream schools, but some have such significant needs that special facilities are provided (see Table 16.2).

'Statementing'

Statementing is an assessment of a child's educational requirements (see Table 16.3). This is started at any time during a child's schooling and is formally reviewed in years 8, 9, 10, and 11 to prepare both the child and the services for action to accommodate the transition to post-school life, whether that is in further education or not. It is a multidisciplinary process and contributions are made by GPs, therapists, nursing staff, social services, teachers, and educational psychologists. The parents have to agree it. As it is reviewed annually, it forms part of a rehabilitation framework for the young person at school, but service inadequacies exist.

Table 16.2 Some comparisons of mainstream versus special schools

Advantages	Disadvantages
Larger schools likely to have better educational facilities	Bigger distances for the disabled child to cover. Increased energy consumption to get around may negate some educational advantages
Likely to have or aspire to higher educational achievement	Disabled child may feel alone in company of able-bodied children in large school
Mixing and competing with the general population	Less understanding of an individual child's overall needs, particularly in time to achieve targets. Child may be seen as a poor achiever
Wider circle of friends	Lack of specialist teachers and specialist aids to teaching
School likely to be nearer than special school	Lack of on-site therapy facilities or therapists
Disability less likely to hinder a child's ability to get on after school	Some facilities may be inaccessible

Table 16.3 Legislation to date

	Date	Action/recommendation
Warnock Report	1978	Critical of state provision and identifying some of the educational special needs
Education Act	1981	Established a statement of children's educational needs. 'Statementing'
Disabled Persons Act, Sections 5 and 6	1986	Important legislation. Identified young people's rights
Education Act	1993	Details of procedures and appeals
Education Act	1996	Refinement of above

Employment

Disabled people in general have high unemployment rates, but only those with cognitive or severe physical problems are incapable of work. Several factors are important, not least the unwillingness (for a number of reasons) of employers to take them on. The cost of lost employment to the nation is enormous and includes direct costs, lost productivity, and reduced services. The longer one is off work, the lower the chance of returning. This falls to around 50%, after 6 months of back pain, to 25% at 1 year and to 10% at 2 years. The commonest medical causes for unemployment are musculoskeletal, mental health, and circulatory disorders:

• Musculoskeletal: 1.78 million workers reporting sick (28% of those on benefits):
  – back pain, 642 000;
  – neck/upper limb problems, 512 000;
  – lower limbs, 212 000;
  – more than one site, 178 000;
  – low back pain: highest incidence in agriculture, construction, food, nursing, and retail industries with 90 million working days lost through spinal disorders (£5–10 billion).

• Mental health disorders account for 20% of sickness benefits payments and are the commonest cause in London. Most are minor problems rather than major psychiatric disease. Many are put down to pressures in the workplace (stress) and may be a reason for this being the second highest cause of health-related premature retirement.

• Circulatory disorders account for 13% of sickness benefits payments. (Prevalence of medical causes of unemployment. British Society of Rehabilitation Medicine Report on Vocational Rehabilitation. 2000. BSRM, London.)

Vocational rehabilitation (VR)

Vocational rehabilitation (see Fig. 16.1) is the concept of enabling temporarily or permanently disabled individuals to access, return, or remain in employment (from the BSRM Report on Vocational Rehabilitation, 2000).

VR schemes have the potential to give a two to ten times return on costs through:
- Reduced sickness absence.
- Reduced early retirement.
- Increased productivity.
- Continued payment of taxes.
- Reduced payment of state benefits.

Team roles in VR
- Rehabilitation Physician: medical and disability assessment, prognostication, medical interventions.
- Occupational therapist: traditionally had a role in returning people to work; well placed to take up this role again (Fig. 16.2).
- Physotherapist: responsible for functional capacity assessment, manual handling education, pre-employment screening, post-injury therapy, risk assessment between workers and work activities, work hardening and work conditioning, workforce health promotion.
- Psychology: emotional and psychological assessments, treatments, e.g. cognitive behavioural therapy.

Fig. 16.1 Schematic view of vocational rehabilitation.

Fig 16.2 Occupational therapy (OT) vocational rehabilitation scheme.

Transition to adult life: the disabled school leaver

The problem

Moving from the relatively well-coordinated facilities of school life to a less structured adult environment can be a major change for people with disabilities and their families (Tables 16.4, 16.5, 16.6). It is a time of great change for us all and young people with disabilities are less equipped to deal with it. On top of this there are organizational changes, and the professional teams that the person and the family were so used to disappear. Paediatricians cease to provide services, and their philosophy of total health care (where children are under the same specialist for acute and on-going health problems) is now replaced by a more fragmented service, where the person and family do not usually get to know their doctor/therapist as well. Disability tends to be higher among ethnic minority groups for whom there are already disadvantages, and is thus a greater burden.

Epidemiology

Table 16.7 outlines the epidemiology of disability in young adults.

Requisite skills for a young adult

The skills required for a young adult to function independently are shown in Table 16.8.

Service provision

Dedicated teams have an advantage over an *ad hoc* approach to service delivery through giving disabled young people better knowledge, information and therefore access to services (Fig. 16.3). They aim to allow the establishment of an adult lifestyle and improve the quality of life of young people with physical disabilities aged between 16 and 25–30 years of age through:

- Healthcare and personal issues—disability, psychosexual, genetic counselling (NHS).
- Equipment for daily living, education, and employment (NHS, social services department (SSD), Department for Education and Science (DfES), Department of Work and Pensions (DWP))
- Information (all agencies).
- Independent living skills (NHS, DfES).
- Social needs, personal care, finance, and occupational activity (NHS, SSD, DWP).
- Further education and training (DfES).
- Transport, mobility and access (all, NHS).
- Housing (local authority).
- Leisure and recreation facilities (SSD, NHS).

Table 16.4 Additional legislation to consider

	Date	Action/recommendation
Disabled Persons Act Sections 5 & 6	1986	Important legislation. Identified the rights of young people
Children's Act	1989	Social services' responsibilities change to adult provision at 19 years
Education Act	1996	Refinement of above
Disability Discrimination Act	1995	Enshrines some disabled person's rights

Table 16.5 Constraints for disabled young adults

Constraint	Examples
Resources	Lack of appropriate facilities
Personal ability	Low self-esteem and self-image
Family concern	Decreased aspirations for child and letting go of childhood
Service mismatching	Failure to match client with facility

Table 16.6 Highlight of mismatch of service provision and individual needs

Lack of coordinated rehabilitation service
Shortage of skilled specialists in health and social services
Poor liaison between services fragmenting response to individuals
Lack of accessible and up-to-date information resource for service users and for providers
Inadequate provision of certain services
Inadequate provision of and lack of choice of residential accommodation
Inadequate day-care provision outside city centres

Table 16.7 Incidence and prevalence of some diseases in young adults

Disease/injury	Incidence per 10^6	Prevalence per 10^6	Prevalence trend
Congenital			
Cerebral palsy	200	—	Static
Spina bifida	Variable	2	Down
Muscular dystrophy— all types	1–3 per 8000 live births	90	Down
Neurological rarities	Make large group together	—	Down
Cystic fibrosis	40/2500 live births	—	Up in >15-year-olds
Acquired			
Head injury	300	150	Up
Spinal injury	10–15	—	Static
Juvenile chronic arthritis	16	<113	Static
Multiple sclerosis	48	99–198	Static

Table 16.8 Skills required of a young adult

	Aspect of life	Specific skills required
Maintenance skills	Health	Nutrition. Exercise. Disease management. Disability management. Use of NHS resources (e.g. GP, dentist)
	Self-care	Feeding, dressing, and hygiene
	Domestic	Food collection, preparation, and storage. Clothes maintenance. Home cleaning/maintenance. Home safety
	Mobility	Indoors, threshold, outdoors. On foot, in wheelchair, using public and private transport
Life skills	Relationships	Sexual, family, social, work, community, other
	Leisure	Hobbies and sport
	Work	Direct work skills and mobility to and within the workplace. Posture and seating
	Self-development	Assertiveness. Negotiation. Time management. Money management. Information aquisition and use. Career development

Fig. 16.3 Links with services.

Multiple sclerosis

Background

Multiple sclerosis (MS) is the commonest cause of severe physical disability in young adults. The progressive and changing nature of the condition combined with the complexity of the resulting disability makes MS one of the most serious challenges to the neurological rehabilitation team. These sections concentrate on the management of disability. Some background details are relevant and are described in the next few sections—epidemiology, natural history, and diagnosis.

Epidemiology

There is a well-known geographical variation in prevalence of MS. There is a strong trend for prevalence to increase with increasing latitude both north and south of the equator. This trend is even noticeable in the UK with lower prevalence rates in the southern part of the country compared with high prevalence rates in the northern Scottish islands—up to 258 per 100 000 population. The overall prevalence rate in the UK is around 120 per 100 000 population. Thus, in the UK a typical general practice with a population of around 2000 will have two to three people with MS on their list.

Incidence in the UK is around 2–6 per 100 000 per annum. In the context of this section it is more relevant to know the proportion of people with MS who are significantly disabled. Around two-thirds of the total MS population is thought to be moderately or severely disabled at any one time. About 80% of people are significantly disabled by 20 years. As the mean age of onset of MS is around 30 it follows that the burden of disability and handicap will fall in the fourth and fifth decades of life.

Natural history and prediction of prognosis

Life expectancy is only modestly shortened in MS. The median survival time is greater than 40 years and as the average age of onset is in the 30s it can be seen there is only a small reduction of life expectancy. There are a few people with rapidly progressive MS who regrettably die within a few years of onset, but such a pattern is unusual. There are a number of different patterns of MS and a few salient points are as follows:

- Two-thirds of people with MS will have a relapsing/remitting course from the onset.
- Around 15% will have a progressive course with superimposed acute episodes.
- The remainder will have a chronically progressive course from onset.
- Most will eventually convert to a progressive course—around 40% by 10 years, 60% by 15 years, and 70% by 25 years.
- The time to conversion to a progressive course is a good predictor of eventual disability—those who become progressive in a short period are more likely to have aggressive disease.
- Around 10% of the MS population do not ever convert to a progressive disease but continue to have relapsing/remitting disease and a benign course.
- It is difficult to predict progression of the disorder. However, the following are generally poor prognostic indicators:
  - Cerebellar symptoms and signs.
  - Polysymptomatic onset.
  - Increasing age of onset—particularly age of onset after 40 years.
  - Onset event giving a disability of greater than 3 on the Kurtzke Disability Status Scale (DSS; see later).
  - Shorter intervals between relapses, particularly less than 1 year.
- Good prognostic signs are:
  - Monosymptomatic onset.
  - Early visual and sensory symptoms.
  - Absence of pyramidal signs 5 years after onset.
  - Absence of cerebellar signs 5 years after onset.
  - Younger age of onset.
  - Initial remitting course.

In the future more accurate prognosis may be possible with more widespread use of serial MRI scanning or by the monitoring of immune markers.

Diagnosis

Diagnosis of MS still rests largely on the traditional clinical skills of history and examination in an attempt to identify clinical lesions of the central nervous system at two or more different anatomical sites that have occurred on at least two separate occasions. Diagnosis is usually assisted or confirmed by:

- Examination of cerebrospinal fluid with evidence of oligoclonal banding and increase in immunoglobulin G production.
- Evoked potential examination.
- Neuroimaging, particularly MRI scanning.

When the history, examination, and investigations are combined MS can be diagnosed with reasonable certainty in the quite early stages. Studies show that the overwhelming majority of people wish to be told the diagnosis at the earliest possible opportunity. This phase of care is still poorly managed and a recent study showed that 10% of people still learnt of their diagnosis by accident or by an incautious remark:

- The diagnosis should be in an unhurried atmosphere, allowing plenty of time for the individual and their family to discuss and ask questions.
- The individual should be given the opportunity for a second appointment soon after the first appointment when further questions have materialized.
- If they wish the individual should be given lay literature regarding MS. There is some particularly good literature produced by the MS Trust and the MS Society in the UK.
- The individual should be put in touch with the local support group who can act in a supportive and counselling role at a time of significant stress and anxiety.

Precipitating and aggravating factors

Pregnancy

The 9 months of pregnancy are a fairly safe time with regard to MS relapse. However, there is a significant increase in relapse rate during the 3–6 months after the birth. Overall pregnancy, or the number of pregnancies, has no effect on subsequent disability. There is also no evidence that the contraceptive pill has any significant influence on the course of the disease.

Stress and life events

There are a number of anecdotal reports of a relationship between emotional shock and onset of the disease. However, more recent work has thrown some doubt on this relationship. Nevertheless, it is still generally accepted that 'extreme' life events, such as a major car accident or divorce, can precipitate a relapse. It is probable that the 'quality' rather than the 'quantity' of stressful life events appears to be the determinant of relapse risk. Obviously the closer the relapse to the stressful event then the more likely is the relationship.

Infection, immunization, and temperature

It is likely that systemic infection can precipitate a relapse but there is little evidence that it can precipitate the onset of MS. It is known that increase of body temperature, such as in a hot bath or after exertion, can be associated with a temporary worsening of symptoms (Uhthoff's phenomenon). There is, other than a few anecdotal reports, little evidence that immunization has any effect on the course of the disease.

Trauma and surgery

The evidence for trauma or surgery having any effect on MS is anecdotal, although there are a few apparently clear-cut cases showing such a relationship. Overall it is generally agreed that:

- There should be a close temporal relationship between the trauma and onset or exacerbation of MS, certainly within 3 months.
- The trauma should actually involve the central nervous system (e.g. brain injury after a road traffic accident).
- Preferably there should be a close anatomical relationship between the presumed site of the MS lesion and the anatomical site of the trauma.

Rating scales

As in all rehabilitation processes it is important for rehabilitation goals to be properly documented. It is probably more valuable to use a particular scale for the symptom that is being treated rather than use an overall disability scale. However, in the MS literature the Kurtzke Expanded Disability Status Scale is very widely used. There are problems with the scale, which mixes impairment with disability, but it is so widely used that it is reproduced in Table 17.1. It is often used in conjunction with a more detailed functional systems scoring, also developed by Kurtzke, but there are other disability scales available (see Chapter 5).

Table 17.1 Kurtzke Expanded Disability Status Scale (EDSS)

Step	Description
0	Normal neurological exam (all grade 0 in functional systems (FS); cerebral grade 1 acceptable)
1.0	No disability, minimal signs in one FS (i.e. grade 1 excluding cerebral grade 1)
1.5	No disability, minimal signs in more than one FS (more than one grade 1 excluding cerebral grade 1)
2.0	Minimal disability in one FS (one FS grade 2, others 0 or 1)
2.5	Minimal disability in two FS (two FS grade 2, others 0 or 1)
3.0	Moderate disability in one FS (one FS grade 3, others 0 or 1), or mild disability in three or four FS (three/four FS grade 2, others 0 or 1) though fully ambulatory
3.5	Fully ambulatory but with moderate disability in one FS (one grade 3) and one or two FS grade 2; or two FS grade 3; or five FS grade 2 (others 0 or 1)
4.0	Fully ambulatory without aid, self-sufficient, up and about some 12 hours a day despite relatively severe disability consisting of one FS grade 4 (others 0 or 1), or combinations of lesser grade exceeding limits of previous steps. Able to walk without aid or rest some 500 m
4.5	Fully ambulatory without aid, up and about much of the day, able to work a full day, may otherwise have some limitation of full activity or require minimal assistance; characterized by relatively severe disability, usually consisting of one FS grade 4 (others 0 or 1) or combinations of lesser grades exceeding limits of previous steps. Able to walk without aid or rest for some 300 m
5.0	Ambulatory without aid or rest for about 200 m; disability severe enough to impair full daily activities (for example, to work a full day without special provisions). (Usual FS equivalents are one grade 5 alone, others 0 or 1; or combinations of lesser grades usually exceeding specifications for step 4.0)
5.5	Ambulatory without aid or rest for about 100 m; disability severe enough to preclude full daily activities. (Usual FS equivalents are one grade 5 alone, others 0 or 1; or combinations of lesser grades usually exceeding specifications for step 4.0)
6.0	Intermittent or unilateral constant assistance (cane, crutch, or brace) required to walk about 100 m with or without resting. (Usual FS equivalents are combinations with more than two FS grade 3+)
6.5	Constant bilateral assistance (canes, crutches, or braces) required to walk about 20 m without resting. (Usual FS equivalents are combinations with more than two FS grade 3+)
7.0	Unable to walk beyond about 5 m even with aid, essentially restricted to wheelchair; wheels self in standard wheelchair and transfers alone; up and about in wheelchair some 12 hours a day. (Usual FS equivalents are combinations with more than one FS grade 4+; very rarely pyramidal grade 5 alone)
7.5	Unable to take more than a few steps; restricted to wheelchair; may need aid in transfer; wheels self but cannot carry on in a standard wheelchair for a full day; may require a motorized wheelchair. (Usual FS equivalents are combinations with more than one FS grade 4+)

Table 17.1 (continued)

Step	Description
8.0	Essentially restricted to bed or chair or perambulated in wheelchair but may be out of bed itself for much of the day; retains many self-care functions; generally has effective use of arms. (Usual FS equivalents are combinations, generally grade 4+ in several systems)
8.5	Essentially restricted to bed much of the day; has some effective use of arm(s); retains some self-care functions. (Usual FS equivalents are combinations, generally 4+ in several systems)
9.0	Helpless bed patient; can communicate and eat. (Usual FS equivalents are combinations, mostly grade 4+)
9.5	Totally helpless bed patient; unable to communicate effectively or eat/swallow. (Usual FS equivalents are combinations, almost all grade 4+)
10	Death due to MS

Disease-modifying treatment

There have recently been significant advances with regard to treatment possibilities for slowing down the progression of MS.

Corticosteroids

Adrenocorticosteroids have been used for many years for the treatment of relapse in MS. The best mode of steroid administration for relapse is intravenous methylprednisolone that can be quite safely given on an out-patient basis and in a single-bolus injection. There is no evidence that long-term steroid treatment has any effect on MS, and indeed it is probably detrimental in terms of undesirable steroid side-effects.

Azathioprine

There is some evidence that this is useful in reducing relapse rate, but is now used less often given the advent of interferon and other more effective therapies.

Cyclophosphamide

Cyclophosphamide is probably efficacious in the progressive phase of the disease, but there is little consensus on a suitable regime. It is associated with significant side-effects.

Glatiramer acetate (Copaxone)

This is a mixture of synthetic basic polypeptides and has recently become available for human use. It is given by daily subcutaneous injection. It is able to reduce the relapse rate and probably has a positive effect on long-term disability. It is usually well tolerated. In the UK there have been problems with prescription which is now restricted to recognized neurological treatment centres.

Interferons

Interferons are a group of naturally occurring proteins that modify the immune response. Interferon gamma appears to stimulate the immune response whereas interferons alpha and beta appear to be immunosuppressants. There have now been good quality and long-term studies that have shown efficacy of alpha and beta interferons in reducing the relapse rate and probably reducing long-term disability. This area has been controversial, and prescription is limited to specific neurological treatment centres. At the moment prescription is also limited to those who have relapsing/remitting disease under certain strict criteria. Each person put on interferon therapy in the UK has to be part of an on-going data collection trial that should confirm, or refute, the efficacy of these treatments over the next few years. The treatments are expensive (around £10 000 per annum per person). All the available compounds require subcutaneous injection. There is a range of troublesome side-effects, including local skin reactions, flu-like symptoms, and headache and a significant minority also seem to develop neutralizing antibodies which effectively stops clinical benefit. The interferons have also been shown to reduce lesion load on MRI scanning, which in theory should mean that there is less accumulating disability over time, but this point is not yet proven.

Other disease-modifying treatments

There have been many treatments that have come and gone in MS. Whilst some may have shown initial promise such promise was not sustained after further studies. Other compounds have shown to have a beneficial effect but are associated with significant side-effects. There are a few therapies worth a brief mention:

- *Hyperbaric oxygen.* This was in vogue in the 1970s but studies failed to support initial enthusiasm, although there may have been some improvement in bladder function and a suggestion of retardation of disease progression.
- *Diet.* The advantage of dietary manipulation is that the individual with MS feels that they are doing something for their own disease. Studies in the 1980s did demonstrate that a diet low in saturated fats and supplemented by N3 polyunsaturated fatty acids showed a non-significant trend towards shorter duration, reduced frequency, and severity of relapses. N3 fatty acids are found in fish oils.

Symptom management

Management of symptoms

There can be few disorders that require so much active interdisciplinary cooperation. The challenge for the rehabilitation team is to manage the complex interaction that lies behind disability, often involving several different neuronal systems. The complexity of the situation is illustrated by Table 17.2 which lists the symptoms in 656 people with MS.

Mobility

Difficulty walking is the most common symptom in MS. It is often due to a combination of different factors including:
- Pyramidal weakness.
- Spasticity.
- Fatigue.
- Disuse.
- Pain.
- Ataxia.
- Proprioceptive problems.

In the early stage a structured exercise programme, planned and supervised by a physiotherapist, can be of benefit. It has been recommended that the elements of such a programme should include:
- Repetition of individual movements in order to increase strength.
- Passive stretching to reduce spasticity, improve the range of movement, and prevent contractures.
- Exercises utilizing activities of daily living to improve dexterity and coordination.
- Gait training using mobility aids as necessary.
- Hydrotherapy to increase activity and range of movement.

It is likely that such an exercise programme will need to be continued for life but the availability of expert physiotherapy is sadly lacking for such long-term monitoring. However, if and when spasticity supervenes then the input of a physiotherapist is vital. The management of spasticity is covered elsewhere (Chapter 6) but the following is a useful list of approaches to treatment:
- Reduction of external stimuli (e.g. catheter repositioning, foot care, bowel management, treatment of skin and urinary infections, etc.).
- Physiotherapy, including hydrotherapy and appropriate use of mobility aids and proper attention to seating and posture, both in wheelchair and leisure seating.
- Dynamic casting and correct use of orthoses.
- Pharmacological management, including peripheral nerve blocks and motor point blocks, botulinum toxin injections, and for more severe cases intrathecal baclofen or orthopaedic and neurosurgical procedures.

If untreated, spasticity can easily lead to muscle contracture which in turn leads to worsening of posture, further pain, and an increased risk of pressure sores.

Upper limb function

Problems with arm functions are often a combination of pyramidal weakness combined with spasticity, ataxia, and sensory disturbance. In the case

Table 17.2 Symptoms in 656 people with multiple sclerosis

Symptom present	No ADL difficulty (%)	With ADL difficulty (%)	Total (%)
Fatigue	21	56	77
Balance problems	24	50	74
Weakness or paralysis	18	45	63
Numbness, tingling, or other sensory disturbance	39	24	63
Bladder problems	25	34	59
Increased muscle tension (spasticity)	23	26	49
Bowel problems	19	20	39
Difficulty remembering	21	16	37
Depression	18	18	36
Pain	15	21	36
Laugh or cry easily (emotional lability)	24	8	32
Double or blurred vision, partial or complete blindness	14	16	30
Shaking (tremor)	14	13	27
Speech and/or communication difficulties	12	11	23
Difficulty solving problems	12	9	21

ADL, activities of daily living.

From Kraft, G.H., Freal, J.E., and Coryll, J.K. (1986). Disability, disease duration and rehabilitation service needs in multiple sclerosis: patient perspectives. *Archives of Physical Medicine and Rehabilitation* **67**: 164–78.

of arm difficulties an occupational therapist will need to be involved. The prescription of appropriate aids to daily living can be immensely helpful both to adapt the environment and for more immediate use by the individual. There is now a remarkable range of simple aids and adaptations that can make hand and arm tasks much simpler. There is some limited evidence that functionally orientated exercises utilizing simple daily living tasks can improve dexterity and coordination. Spasticity treatment in the arm is much more difficult than the leg, as the arm is less accessible to peripheral nerve blocks and much less amenable to surgical intervention.

Cerebellar dysfunction
Regrettably cerebellar involvement is common and also difficult to treat. There is little convincing evidence of a reliable improvement using any treatment. Specific drugs can sometimes be used with limited success, including:
- Isoniazid.
- Choline.

Symptom management (*continued*)

- Benzodiazepines.
- Sodium valproate.

Functional improvement will usually rest on the provision of adaptive equipment, such as:
- Weighted bands on the wrists.
- Large-handled implements.
- Plate guards.
- Velcro fastenings for buttons and shoelaces.
- Electric toothbrushes.
- Electric page turners, etc.

Occasionally severe intention tremor can be treated by cryothalamotomy or more recently by deep brain stimulation. Sometimes botulinum toxin can reduce very severe intention tremor but at the risk of generalized weakness.

Swallowing disorders

Fortunately swallowing disorders are not that common except in very late stage MS. Swallowing disorders have been covered in Chapter 9. In summary it is now recognized that swallowing is a highly complex motor sequence that requires expert evaluation by a speech therapist, dietician, and radiographer. Videofluoroscopy is really the only way to make a proper assessment of dysphagia. However, there are a number of treatment possibilities for the different types of dysphagia. In later stage MS there is often an ethical problem with regard to swallowing disorders. How active should management be? In the author's view if, despite dietary manipulation, there are still difficulties with oral feeding and risk of malnutrition then a percutaneous endoscopic gastrostomy (PEG) tube should be considered sooner rather than later. This is a benign procedure and will usually improve quality of life.

Communication problems

Dysphasia is quite unusual in MS. The main problems of communication arise from dysarthria. Early referral to a speech therapist is important as there is evidence that early referral can improve functional communication abilities. Fortunately less than 1% of people with MS require augmentative communication aids but it is important to recognize the significant improvement in quality of life that can follow the prescription of such aids in this minority.

Continence

Urinary problems are very common in MS. Urinary difficulties probably account for more handicap than any other problem. The commonest symptoms are:
- Urgency.
- Urge incontinence.
- Frequency.

These symptoms tend to be associated with bladder over-activity (detrusor hyper-reflexia). However, symptoms are not a reliable means of determining the underlying pathophysiology and urodynamics should be undertaken. About half the people with MS who have detrusor hyper-reflexia are also shown to have detrusor sphincter dyssynergia (see Chapter 7).

Less common symptoms are those often associated with bladder hypo-activity:

- Hesitancy.
- Overflow incontinence.
- Use of abdominal pressure when voiding.
- Episodes of retention.

These symptoms occur in about a quarter of those with MS with urinary symptoms.

Involvement of the upper urinary tract should now be unusual if there has been proper monitoring and urological follow-up. Whilst urodynamic assessment is important it is probably reasonable to offer anti-cholinergic medication on an empirical basis in the first instance if someone presents with frequency, urgency, and occasional urge incontinence. First choice is probably oxybutynin (dose 2.5–3 mg twice a day increasing to a maximum of 5 mg three times a day). Other possibilities are Probanthine and imipramine. If this medication is not sufficient then urodynamic assessment is required.

Intermittent catheterization has markedly improved management for many people. Residual post-micturition volume should be ascertained, preferably by ultrasound, although post-micturition catheterization is a reasonable alternative. If the residual volume is over 100 ml this is probably an indication for catheterization. Intermittent catheterization either by the patient or by a third party is the first choice. However, weakness, incoordination, adductor spasticity, or unavailability of a suitable carer can still necessitate an indwelling catheter. Suprapubic catheterization has been shown to be much safer, with less risk of infection, than urethral catheterization.

Most people are able to manage their urinary symptoms by a combination of anti-cholinergic medication and intermittent catheterization—only around 10% need more specialist urological referral and treatment. Appropriate use should be made of the specialist nurse continence advisors that are now widely available throughout the UK. These individuals can provide practical advice on aids and appliances as well as psychological support and counselling.

Bowel problems

Constipation can occur in many people with MS. Fortunately faecal incontinence is less common, although faecal overflow can occur in the context of constipation. The situation is usually resolved by:

- Attention to both timing and amount of time spent in defaecation.
- Maximal use of gastric colic reflex.
- Appropriate use of mechanical factors, such as hip flexion during defaecation.
- Abdominal pressure or digital stimulation can be helpful.
- A diet high in fibre supplemented, if needed, by bulking agents with adequate water intake.
- If the above measures fail then other medication can be used, such as sodium docusate, laxatives, and enemas.

Symptom management (*continued*)

Sexual function

In one study three-quarters of the men and over half of the women had sexual problems in the context of MS. In women this mainly was secondary to:

- Fatigue.
- Decreased sensation.
- Decreased libido.
- Problems with orgasm.

In men fatigue and decreased libido were also problems but they also had difficulty in achieving and maintaining erection.

The management of sexual difficulties is a specialist field and if possible referral to an appropriate sexual advisory service for people with disabilities should be made. Sexual counselling and treatment can consist of the following:

- Straightforward practical advice, such as the best time for intercourse with regard to fatigue.
- Optimization of medication.
- Correct advice on bladder management.
- Advice on positioning.

Adductor spasticity can be a particular problem which may be helped by physiotherapy or nerve blocks. Erectile dysfunction in the male is now usually treated by sildenafil (Viagra). If Viagra cannot be tolerated then male erectile dysfunction can be helped by self-injection of papavarine. Other techniques include vacuum condom and venostricture devices and sometimes the use of penile prostheses, but the latter techniques have now been largely superseded by the use of Viagra.

The main point to emphasize is for sexuality to be viewed in its broadest context—only part of which is penetrative sexual intercourse.

There is no evidence that fertility is impaired in MS.

Pain and paroxysmal symptoms

Pain can be a real difficulty in MS. Around half of people have an acute or chronic pain problem. Some people have acute paroxysmal pain including:

- Trigeminal neuralgia.
- L'Hermitte's syndrome (pain on neck flexion).
- Paroxysmal burning pain.
- Painful tonic seizures.

These paroxysmal painful syndromes respond well to anti-convulsant medication such as carbamazepine or gabapentin.

Longer-term pain can be due to a variety of causes, including:

- Musculoskeletal pain secondary to posture disturbance, such as wheelchair dependency giving rise to low back pain or shoulder pain secondary to self-propelling of the wheelchair.
- Chronic neuralgic pain, probably secondary to the disease process itself—this can respond to carbamazepine and/or gabapentin.
- Pain from spasticity, which can respond to anti-spastic measures, particularly botulinum toxin; this can also act as an analgesic as well as an anti-spastic agent.

Visual disturbance

Optic neuritis is one of the main presenting symptoms of MS and will often respond well to corticosteroid therapy. However, there are a range of other problems including:
- Residual scotomas.
- Diplopia.
- Oscillopsia.

Many such symptoms are difficult to treat. Symptomatic nystagmus can be helped by converging prisms or botulinum toxin therapy. Referral to low-vision clinics can sometimes be necessary and helpful.

General medical problems

There are a whole variety of other general medical difficulties that can arise in MS. These would include:
- Pressure sores.
- Peripheral oedema.
- Deep venous thrombosis (but fortunately people with MS seem to have a low risk).
- Heterotopic ossification (but also rare in MS).
- Hearing problems (very rare in MS).

Fatigue

This is the commonest symptom in MS. It can have an overwhelming effect on daily activities and may be the main reason for handicap in terms of employment and leisure interests. The fatigue in MS can be secondary to depression or to the high energy cost of walking or other daily tasks. However, it seems that there is also a direct central mechanism for MS-related fatigue as there is only a poor correlation between fatiguability and physical disability.

Management of fatigue depends on:
- Frequent rest periods throughout the day.
- Attention to sleep problems that may reduce daytime fatigue, such as the cautious and judicious use of short-acting benzodiazepines. The principle of 'little and often' is often the best way of managing fatigue.
- The use of anti-fatigue agents, such as amantadine, can also be helpful.

Cognitive dysfunction

Intellectual impairment was recognized by the earliest describers of MS, such as Charcot and l'Hermitte. In modern practice cognitive problems have tended to be under-emphasized. However, there is no doubt that cognitive impairment can be detected even in the early stages of MS. The commonest problems are:
- Memory difficulties.
- Problems with information processing speed—the individual may appear 'slow on the uptake'.
- Retrograde learning.

Some recommend brief screening tests, such as the Mini Mental State Examination or the Screening Examination for Cognitive Impairment (SEFCI), which can be useful as an aid to deciding who to refer to for

Symptom management (*continued*)

a more complete neuropsychological assessment. Preferably a clinical neuropsychologist should be an integral part of any MS rehabilitation team.

Emotional problems

Depression occurs in up to 50% of the MS population at some point. There is no evidence that depression in the context of MS responds any differently from other depressive illness and should be treated appropriately (see Chapter 14).

Clinical anxiety is a further problem which is often made worse by lack of proper information or time for simple counselling and support. The MS literature refers to euphoria being quite common, although this does seem to be a most unusual symptom.

A small number of people develop emotionalism (see Chapter 14) which responds well to a small dose of a tricyclic anti-depressant.

Participation issues

Problems in MS can often be unnecessarily compounded by a lack of knowledge regarding local services and facilities. Health professionals in the rehabilitation team should be acquainted with:

- Local accessible leisure pursuits.
- Day centre provision.
- Respite care provision.
- How to access local housing and housing adaptation systems.
- Welfare rights services.
- Employment rehabilitation services.
- Carer support groups.
- Information and advice services.
- Contact address of local and national MS societies and other self-help groups.

It is particularly important to emphasize employment rehabilitation. This can be a major concern amongst the MS population as the disease mainly affects those of working age. About 80% of the economic loss to the national economy from people with MS is accounted for by lost earnings. The unemployment rate in most studies is very high and usually exceeds 50%.

Service delivery

There is now good evidence that access to a skilled multidisciplinary rehabilitation team can make a real impact on the lives of people with MS. Studies have shown that a brief period (around 2 weeks) of inpatient admission to a rehabilitation unit can reduce disability and handicap even in the context of worsening impairment. However, it is probable that such benefits may be lost over time if there is no long-term support. Individuals with MS should preferably have access to the rehabilitation team on a regular basis—even if this just involves simple telephone advice or self-referral at times of problems. A formal regular review is probably needed in order to prevent unnecessary or unrecognized complications from arising. Evidence in Newcastle upon Tyne showed that the costs of introducing a community-based MS team were matched by the reduction in costs from unnecessary hospital admissions, outpatient referrals, and reduction in GP contact time.

The needs of the MS family focus on the following:

- Time—to discuss diagnosis and treatment as well as more personal cognitive and emotional difficulties. A counsellor attached to the MS team is a valuable asset.
- Information—at the time of diagnosis and in the longer term to keep up to date with research and potential treatments.
- Practical help—in terms of the provision of aids and equipment as well as access to personal help within the home.
- Carers need—an equal need for access to information and counselling support as well as the need for access to respite facilities.

The recent development of a network of MS nurse specialists has been a welcome addition to community support. The nurses are well trained and can deal with many daily problems in MS and also act as a source of referral to more specialist support. Every individual with MS should have access to an MS nurse specialist and preferably access to a specialist rehabilitation team.

Chapter 18

Stroke

Definition and epidemiology

A stroke is an insult to the brain as a result of a cerebrovascular accident, in which there is an interruption to the normal cerebral circulation resulting in the onset of neurological loss over a short period of time. This follows either an intracerebral haemorrhage, a cerebral infarction, or a subarachnoid haemorrhage. Transient cerebral ischaemic attack (or mini-stroke) is defined by symptoms lasting for not more than 24 h. There is a need to distinguish these three because there are different factors in primary and secondary prevention and some differing rehabilitative needs. Subarachnoid haemorrhage (in contrast to cerebral infarction and haemorrhage) often presents with more global deficits producing significant cognitive as well as physical problems. There is agreement that early intervention does bring benefits, both in terms of mortality and morbidity (Table 18.1).

Table 18.1 Epidemiology of stroke

Incidence	Common: 200/100 000 population
Prevalence	550/100 000 population, 400 with significant disability per 250 000 population
Mortality	30% in first month, 40% in first year. Myocardial infarction, bronchopneumonia, and further stroke are the commonest causes
Disability	50% weakness, 15–20% dysphasia, 10% cognitive deficit (memory, perception, intellect, and other higher cerebral functioning)

Classification and diagnosis

Stroke can be classified as follows:
- Transient ischaemic attack.
- Subarachnoid haemorrhage
- Intracerebral haemorrhage
- Infarction:
  - Total anterior circulation infarct.
  - Partial anterior circulation infarct.
  - Lacunar infarct.
  - Posterior circulation infarct.

The impairments resulting from stroke depend on the location of the lesion.

Lacunar infarcts

These are often multiple and result from occlusion of small arteries of 50–150 mm in diameter. They are associated with hypertension and arteriosclerosis and give rise to multiple deep small cavities, known as lacunae. They produce four specific syndromes which are as follows:
- Hemiparesis with ataxia affecting the leg more than the arm (from an infarct in the internal capsule).
- Pure motor hemiplegia (from an infarct in the pons or internal capsule).
- Dysarthric–clumsy hand syndrome (pons)—dysarthria, slight dysphagia, central facial weakness, deviation of tongue to the affected side, and clumsiness and ataxia in the ipsilateral hand to the side of lesion.
- Pure sensory stroke with unilateral sensory loss for all modalities of sensation (posterolateral thalamic nucleus infarct).

Rarer syndromes, e.g. lateral medullary syndromes, can be found in more detail in a neurology text.

Anatomy and localizing features of brain disease

Impairments/deficits depending on the site of the lesion are shown in Table 18.2. Visual loss is illustrated in Fig. 18.1.

Table 18.2 Impairment/deficit according to the site of the brain lesion

Site of lesion	Impairment/deficit
Frontal lobe	Behavioural abnormalities. Planning/anticipatory difficulties. Inertia and decreased initiative
Parietal lobe	Spatial disorientation. Apraxia. Agnosia. Sensory inattention. **Receptive dysphasia. *Homonymous hemianopia
Pre-central gyrus (in parietal lobe)	Localized weakness/monoplegia. *Expressive dysphasia
Post-central gyrus	Localized sensory loss
Temporal lobe	Memory. Hallucination (auditory and visual). Decreased concentration/attention. Receptive dysphasia. Quadratic hemianopia
Occipital lobe	Hemianopia
Base of brain	Hemiplegia and hemi-anaesthesia. Spasticity++ cranial nerve deficits
Brainstem	Ataxia. Cranial nerve problems, particularly dysarthria and diplopia. Spasticity+++ diffuse (as found in SAH). Decreased information processing. Decreased IQ. Cognitive problems

* Dominant hemisphere. ** Non-dominant hemisphere. SAH, subarachnoid haemorrhage.

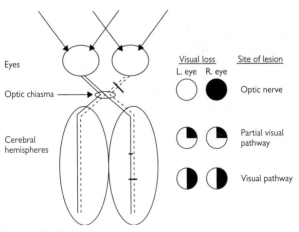

Fig. 18.1 Visual loss in stroke.

Investigations

The completed stroke
- Urgent CT scans are performed to determine the site and size of the lesion. CT scans are normal in about 15% of cases. They actually rarely change the management of the patient, but are essential in four specific situations:
    - To exclude cerebral haemorrhage when anti-coagulant or anti-platelet treatment is being considered.
    - When there is a suspicion that a patient has an intracranial mass due to tumour, subdural haematoma, or abscess.
    - When intracranial hypertension is suspected, particularly if the patient's level of consciousness is dropping and surgical intervention is being considered.
    - When the patient's course is atypical and the diagnosis is in doubt.
- All other investigations are directed to:
    - excluding other causes of the acute stroke syndrome;
    - revealing some underlying cause for the stroke; or
    - detecting some potential complication of a stroke.
- Differential:
    - Tumours/subdural haematoma: seek surgical advice.
    - Post-epileptic paresis: non-specific change in consciousness.
    - Biochemical abnormalities: require investigation—rarely cause stroke.
    - Myocardial disease: cardiac assessment is important; anti-coagulants for atrial fibrillation in absence of cerebral haemorrhage.

Transient ischaemic attacks (TIAs)
- TIAs require full investigation in order to prevent completed strokes. Management centres on reducing the risk factors (hypertension, smoking, diabetes, and other rarer abnormalities, e.g. anaemia, polycythaemia).
- Look for: arrhythmias, significant carotid artery occlusion (treatable by endarterectomy), reducing risk factors by health education (cessation of smoking, weight reduction in obese people, lipid reduction, diabetic control, and increasing physical activity).

Rehabilitation of the completed stroke patient

There is no such thing as a 'simple stroke', since neither the disabilities nor the patient's circumstances are ever straightforward. Each patient needs individual consideration within a standard plan for assessment.

Medical assessment

A comprehensive history (which may have to be provided by a relative in patients with communication or cognitive problems) and examination to identify impairments, functioning, and potential for participation:

- Physical and nutritional status.
- Motor and sensory deficits, including visual field defects, dysaesthesia, and paraesthesiae.
- Incontinence.
- Tissue viability problems.
- Spasticity.
- Dysphagia (due to poor bulbar function).
- Communication difficulties.
- Cognitive deficits and mood.
- The patient's domestic situation and social history.
- The health of carers and their ability to carry out care functions.
- Pre-existing and co-morbid disease, which may act as a barrier to successful rehabilitation.

Predictors of prognostication

Table 18.3 sets out the main prognostic indicators. Social circumstances (socio-economic class, wealth, home ownership, and a good supportive family) can affect the chance of a patient living at home, but they are not, somewhat strangely, indicators *per se* of a good prognosis in terms of independent living. Good cognition and communication and the ability to move the thumb and the foot are better.

Table 18.3 Prognostic indicators in stroke

Early mortality at onset	Capillary abnormalities. Gaze paresis. Abnormal respiratory pattern. Bilateral extensor plantar responses. Persistence of hypertension and significant cardiac disease
Poor signs at 1 week	MRC grade 0 power in upper limb. Unable to locate affected thumb with eyes closed. Cannot maintain sitting balance. Incontinence. Loss of consciousness at onset
4-week prognosticators of poor functional outcome	Low scores in the Barthel scale of activities of daily living (ADL). Pre-existing and post-stroke incontinence
Adverse factors	Inability to walk. Loss of arm function. Loss of postural control. Hemianopia. Proprioceptive sensory loss. Spatial neglect. Impaired cognition
Rate limiting barriers in rehabilitation	Pre-existing physical disability (e.g. joint or cardiopulmonary disease). Multiple pathology (e.g. loss of limb). Sensory impairment. Complications of disabling disease. Incontinence. Pressure sores. Impairment of intellect, memory, perception, communication, and mood
Signs for good outcome	Reverse of poor signs. Early return of hand movement and shoulder protraction (return of prehensile function and ADL). Youth, and a motivation to achieve realistic targets

Special points in assessment

History taking and examination are important, not only for identifying prognostic factors, but for providing medical input into the rehabilitation process. The following headings are suggested:
- Motor function.
- Swallowing.
- Vision.
- Communication.
- Higher cerebral functions.
- Sensation.
- Other problems.

Formal measurement is important and this is addressed in Chapter 5.

Motor function

Assess dexterity and shoulder function, the ability to initiate movements, grip, pinch grip, ability to raise the hand to the mouth or occiput, walking speed (10 m walking time), and Ashworth score.

Swallowing

Time taken to drink 150 ml of water. If there is any choking, the test should be aborted immediately and suction should always be at hand to deal with any problems. People with normal swallowing functions can usually manage this quantity of fluid within 10 to 12 s.

Vision

Formal visual field testing by perimetry should be undertaken when visual loss is suspected.

Communication

See Chapter 10.

Higher cerebral functions

See Table 18.4.

Special problems

These include:
- Incontinence, constipation and pressure sores.
- Pressure sores. Check the skin regularly.
- Side-effects of medical treatments.
- Spasticity is a major issue in stroke.
- Depression.

Table 18.4 Assessment of higher cerebral functions after stroke

Cognitive disorder	Appropriate bedside test
Orientation	Hodkinson's test
Memory	Mini Mental State Examination
Perception	Rivermead Behavioural Inattention Test (star cancellation, line crossing)
Apraxia—ideomotor	Miming simple action, e.g. whistling, combing hair, smiling, waving
Apraxia—ideational	More complex tasks such as miming, lighting candle or cigarette, opening door
Apraxia—constructional	Drawings, building blocks etc. (pick five standard tasks for each problem and simple scores can be derived)
Numeracy and intellect	Serial sevens—subtraction from 100. Require detailed thorough examination by a clinical psychologist, e.g. IQ, using WAIS-R scale

Suggested further reading

1 Warlow, C.P., Dennis, M.S., Van Gijn, K., et al. (2001). *Stroke: A Practical Guide to Management.* Blackwell Science, Oxford.

2 Wade, D. (1992). *Measurement in Neurological Disability.* Oxford University Press, Oxford.

Traumatic brain injury

Background and epidemiology

Head injury is one of the most challenging disorders faced by the rehabilitation team. An individual with traumatic brain injury will often have a complex range of physical, behavioural, emotional, cognitive, and social problems. However, there is now good evidence that a multidisciplinary rehabilitation team can make a real difference to outcome and that such a team is clearly preferable to management on a general medical or surgical ward. Regrettably few people in the UK or elsewhere in the world yet have access to such a team. Most people receive good-quality immediate neurosurgical care but most are then discharged back to the local district general hospital or straight back home without any rehabilitation support or follow-up. There are now a few regional specialist neurological rehabilitation centres that cater for such individuals but they are still insufficient to cater for the needs of all those with severe brain injury, let alone those with moderate or milder problems. More importantly there are virtually no good quality community head injury teams that work with the person after the acute phase when they have returned home.

The annual attendance rate at casualty departments with a traumatic brain injury is around 1500–2000 per 100 000 population per annum. Obviously the majority of these people have a minor head injury. Around 10% have a moderate head injury and about 5% a severe head injury. Formal definition of these categories is give in Table 19.1.

The majority of brain injuries are secondary to road traffic accidents, with a smaller proportion due to domestic or industrial accidents, sporting injuries, or violence. Prevalence is thought to be around 100–150 individuals with persistent disability as a result of traumatic brain injury per 100 000 population.

Table 19.1 Classification of head injury

Classification	Definition
Mild head injury	Glasgow Coma Score 13 or 14 or coma <15 min
Moderate head injury	Glasgow Coma Score 8–12 with coma between 15 min and 6 h or post-traumatic amnesia <24 h
Severe head injury	Glasgow Coma Score <7 or coma >6 h or post-traumatic amnesia >24 h

Glasgow Coma Scale

The Glasgow Coma Scale is the most well-known scale. It probably reflects the severity of brain injury and there is a correlation between the Glasgow Coma Scale score and eventual outcome. Obviously the lower the score the worse the eventual outcome. The Glasgow Coma Scale is given in Table 19.2.[1–3]

Table 19.2 Glasgow Coma Scale[1-3]

Item	Response	Score	Details
Eye opening	None	1	Even to pain (supra-orbital pressure)
	To pain	2	Pain from sternum/limb/supra-orbital ridge pressure
	To speech	3	Non-specific response, not necessarily to command
	Spontaneous	4	Eyes open, not necessarily aware
Motor response	None	1	To any pain; limbs remain flaccid
	Extension	2	'Decerebrate'; shoulder adducted and internally rotated, forearm pronated
	Abnormal flexion	3	'Decorticate'; shoulder flexes/adducts
	Withdrawal	4	Arm withdraws from pain, shoulder abducts
	Localizes pain	5	Arm attempts to remove supra-orbital/chest pressure
	Obeys commands	6	Follows simple commands
Verbal response	None	1	As stated
	Incomprehensible	2	Moans/groans; no words
	Inappropriate	3	Intelligible, no sustained sentences
	Confused	4	Responds with conversation, but confused
	Oriented	5	Aware of time, place, person

Prognosis

There is no accurate way of determining prognosis in traumatic brain injury. Certain clear generalizations are possible:

- The lower the initial Glasgow Coma Scale the worse the outcome.
- The longer the coma the worse the outcome.
- The longer the period of post-traumatic amnesia the worse the outcome. (The latter is defined as the period of time from injury until resumption of day-to-day memory.)
- There is a crude correlation between the amount of brain damage (as determined by MRI scanning) and long-term outlook.

However, there are many exceptions to these general rules and it is always unwise to give any definite prognosis within the first few weeks of injury.

Most physical recovery will occur in the first 12 months, but some physical improvement can certainly occur during the second year after injury. Neuropsychological recovery takes much longer and between 2 and 3 years is usually taken as a reasonable length of time for natural recovery to continue. After this period of time, once natural recovery has been completed, functional improvements can still occur by development of appropriate coping strategies and support mechanisms.

Life expectancy is usually normal after head injury except for people with severe disabilities. There are generally agreed to be five factors that reduce life expectancy in traumatic brain injury and indeed in the disabled population as a whole. These are:

- Immobility.
- Incontinence.
- Inability to swallow and consequent necessity of tube or percutaneous endoscopic gastrostomy (PEG) feeding.
- On-going and uncontrolled epilepsy.
- Severe cognitive and intellectual damage.

There are some early indications that after traumatic brain injury individuals may have a higher risk of dementia in later life. However, this is still controversial and such a link is by no means definite.

Minor head injury

The great majority of people with a minor, or even a moderate, head injury make an excellent recovery over a few days or after a week or so. However, there is a significant minority (probably around 10%) of people with minor head injury who continue to have long-term problems over many months or even in the long term. In the past such symptoms have been called 'post-concussional' but such a blanket label is probably best avoided. It is better to annotate each separate symptom in order to determine whether anything can be done about each individual problem. Some of the commoner 'post-concussional' symptoms are:

- Headaches.
- Dizziness.
- Insomnia.
- Fatigue.
- Poor concentration.
- Mild memory disturbance/forgetfulness.
- Slowed ability to learn and process new information.
- Anxiety.
- Depression.
- Irritability.
- Sleep disturbance.

These problems can be cumulative following repeated minor head injury, which may account for some of the longer-term problems encountered in, for example, boxing or horse racing.

It is now generally accepted that such problems are organic in nature rather than related to psychological factors such as coping style or symptom exaggeration in the context of litigation.

In an ideal world everyone with a minor head injury should be followed up at least once after around 3 months in order to identify those who are more likely to have persistent problems. Those individuals may need longer-term counselling and support or perhaps specific interventions, such as full neuropsychological assessment and a cognitive remediation programme.

It is likely that symptoms can be reduced by proper information being given at the time of the head injury at discharge from casualty. A series of booklets on head injury, and in particular mild head injury, produced by the Headway charity are useful in this regard. Contact could be made with the local Headway group for further peer support.

It is regrettably common that people with minor head injury return to work too soon and find that they have difficulty coping with their job. Proper information and advice, not only to the head-injured person but also the employer and the person's family, is vital.

Regrettably there are very few mild head injury clinics in the UK or indeed worldwide.

Organization of services

There are a number of stages to proper care of individuals after traumatic brain injury.

Stage 1: Immediate trauma care

Fast emergency care and appropriate road-side treatment are important followed by rapid transfer to the nearest trauma centre for stabilization. Such centres should be in close association with the neurosurgical unit with access to MRI scanning and cerebral pressure monitoring. Occasionally neurosurgical intervention will be necessary for evacuation of blood clots, elevation of depressed skull fracture, etc. The rehabilitation team should be associated with the acute neurosurgical team. There are a number of complications that can arise in the first few hours and days after injury which if dealt with properly can prevent major rehabilitation difficulties later. An example would be active intervention for spasticity in order to prevent contractures, and assessment of swallowing with appropriate initiation of gastrostomy feeding.

Stage 2: Post-acute rehabilitation

As soon as the individual is surgically and medically stable they should be transferred to the nearest specialist head injury rehabilitation centre. Regrettably there are few such centres in the UK and many people bypass this stage. There is now clear evidence that post-acute brain injury rehabilitation produces better functional outcome. The sooner the transfer is made to the rehabilitation unit the better the outcome.

Stage 3: 'Step-down' rehabilitation

Most people with severe brain injury will make rapid progress over the first few months after the accident. However, after around 6 months progress will begin to plateau. At this time they still have further rehabilitation potential and sometimes transfer to a 'step-down' rehabilitation unit is appropriate. This is a step towards discharge home and such a unit may concentrate on smooth staged discharge back into the home environment. Such a unit is usually most appropriate when there are delays to being transferred home, such as the need for home adaptations. Alternatively individuals with severe cognitive and intellectual damage or behavioural disturbance may need a much more prolonged period of rehabilitation in a less acute environment. Many individuals will bypass this stage and move straight back home.

Stage 4: Community-based rehabilitation

Obviously it is the eventual aim that everyone returns home after traumatic brain injury. Sometimes this is not possible, but nevertheless the great majority of people should be able to get back to their home and family. There is good evidence that the most significant problems for the family and carers occur after discharge home and at this stage long-term support is essential. This should consist of on-going home-based rehabilitation by a multidisciplinary team. Often a care manager is required to coordinate the complex range of services that are required. Physiotherapists, occupational therapists, speech and language therapists, clinical psychologists, medical staff, and social service staff can still need to be involved. Long-term emotional support both to the disabled person and the family is often required. Regrettably there are few coordinated community based rehabilitation teams in the UK or elsewhere.

Thus, there are regrettably very few people who go through a proper staged rehabilitation process after traumatic brain injury. This is a pity as there is now good evidence of the efficacy of a staged multidisciplinary rehabilitation programme.

Each stage should not be seen as a self-contained entity as liaison will still be needed between the staff in the acute rehabilitation unit and, for example, the community team. Staff sharing is often appropriate. Sometimes individuals will need referral back to a specialist centre for management of particular problems, such as PEG feeding or spasticity management. Occasionally referral needs to be made to a specialist subunit, such as a unit catering for people with severe behavioural disturbance.

Physical disability

Severe physical disability following brain injury is quite uncommon. The brain appears to have a remarkable capacity for functional recovery even after quite severe injury. However, a whole range of physical problems are obviously possible after brain trauma. The commonest problems are:

- Walking problems—usually secondary to either spasticity, weakness, or ataxia but often there is a multifactorial causation (see Chapter 6).
- Problems with daily living tasks secondary to similar difficulties in the arms.
- Communication problems secondary to dysarthria or dysphasia (see Chapter 10).
- Swallowing problems often secondary to brainstem damage. PEG feeding is commonly required in severe brain injury at least for the first few months (see Chapter 9).
- Continence problems—usually secondary to detrusor hyper-reflexia or sometimes to detrusor sphincter dyssynergia (see Chapter 7).
- Visual disturbance—blindness, diplopia, or visual neglect.
- Sensory disturbance often compounded by sensory neglect, although this is more common after focal cerebral lesions, such as stroke.
- Loss of the sense of smell is very common even in minor head injuries.
- Post-traumatic epilepsy (see below).

Obviously many of these problems are amenable to rehabilitation intervention. Treatment for these various symptoms are described in other chapters of this book.

Post-traumatic epilepsy

Epilepsy after traumatic brain injury is more common if:

- There is a depressed skull fracture.
- There has been intracranial haemorrhage.
- There is clear focal brain damage as opposed to diffuse axonal injury.
- Later epilepsy is common if there has been an epileptic seizure within the first week after injury.

There are tables that indicate the risk of epilepsy according to the presence or absence of these risk factors. If no risk factors are present then the risk of post-traumatic epilepsy is relatively small at only about 2–3%. Many authorities would not initiate prophylactic anti-convulsant medication unless there is a very high risk of epilepsy. Carbamazepine is probably the anti-convulsant of first choice in epilepsy secondary to traumatic brain injury.

Coma and the vegetative state

Around 1% of people after head injury remain in a prolonged coma (defined as a coma of more than 2 weeks' duration). About half of those who remain in a coma at 1 month have regained consciousness by 3 months although overall functional outlook for this group remains poor. Less than 10% of those recovering from coma that has lasted up to 3 months return to any form of employment. The longer individuals remain comatose the poorer the outcome. Life expectancy is clearly reduced in those with prolonged coma, although there are cases of individuals surviving many years in such a state. Survival is usually dependent on continuing high-quality nursing care, particularly avoidance of pressure sores and active treatment of infections as well as continuing nutrition, usually by PEG feeding.

There is some, very limited, evidence that sensory stimulation can shorten the duration of coma, and despite the lack of hard evidence many centres do promote the use of multisensory stimulation techniques, including touch, smell, taste, and visual stimulation.

Difficult ethical issues arise when the treating rehabilitation team and the family are agreed that active treatment should be withdrawn. In the UK such decisions are now taken by the Court. The family and the treating physician will need to be in agreement. An independent medical expert is appointed both for the patient and also for the hospital and family. Solicitors are also appointed on both sides in order to make sure there is no major financial advantage that would accrue to a third party following the patient's death. The expert reports are presented to a judge who will make a final decision. Euthanasia remains illegal in most countries but withdrawal of active treatment, such as withdrawal of feeding, is allowable after appropriate Court approval.

Great care must be taken in making a diagnosis of persistent or permanent vegetative state. One study indicated a misdiagnosis rate of 40%. Some individuals seem to retain some awareness which is difficult to access and only becomes apparent after detailed and prolonged observation. Deafness and/or visual problems also seem quite common in those with prolonged coma which makes proper assessment even more difficult. The quality of life of people in prolonged coma is probably maximized by transfer to a specialist coma unit. Regrettably there are very few such units in the UK or worldwide.

Cognitive problems

There are a large variety of important cognitive and intellectual problems that follow traumatic brain injury. The assessment and treatment of these conditions is covered in more detail in Chapter 15. The commonest problems are:

- Problems with recent memory.
- Difficulties with concentration and attention.
- Slowed learning speed and reduced information-processing speed.
- Poor initiation.
- Difficulties with planning, often needing someone else to prompt and guide the person even for simple daily living tasks.
- Problem solving.
- Perceptual problems—often visual or sensory neglect.
- Problems with topographical orientation and naming problems.
- Communication problems, particularly dysphasia and dysarthria.

Rehabilitation depends on accurate assessment, which should be carried out by a clinical neuropsychologist. Such assessment needs to not only document the areas of impairment but also the areas of relatively intact function which can be used to form an appropriate coping strategy.

There is now emerging evidence that various cognitive strategies can produce improvements in quality of life and real functional improvements in the clinic setting can generalize back at home. Some brain injury rehabilitation units now have specific cognitive clinics where such people can be assessed and coping strategies planned and enacted.

The use of simple memory aids, diaries, pagers, and the use of mnemonics can, for example, produce significant benefit for those with memory problems (see Chapter 15).

Behavioural and emotional problems

Behavioural problems

Behavioural problems are very common in the early recovery phase following brain injury. At this stage sedative and psychotropic medication should be avoided if at all possible. Such drugs simply add to the confusion and general clouding of consciousness. This in turn can cause more behavioural disturbance leading to a vicious circle. At this stage individuals are often best nursed in separate rooms with quiet surroundings and lack of sensory stimulation. Some brain injury units now have a post-traumatic amnesia (PTA) room in order to nurse such people.

A small number of people after brain injury develop longer-term behavioural difficulties which can amount to significant verbal and physical aggression. Behavioural management techniques are known to be effective in ameliorating such problems. Such techniques are often best put into place in specialist units so that all staff and relatives can cooperate in a strict behavioural regime. The nature of behavioural management programmes has been described in Chapter 13.

Emotional problems

After brain injury it is common to hear relatives complain that 'he is not the person I married' or 'it is like living with a different person'. However, the term 'personality change' should be avoided. It is better to document the details of any perceived change in order that appropriate strategies can be designed to alleviate the problem. There are many such changes and the commonest are:

- Childish or fatuous behaviour.
- Egocentricity.
- Irritability.
- Aggression.
- Lack of initiation and reduced drive.
- Lethargy.
- Lack of social skills.
- Increased or decreased sexual interest.

These problems cause family and work disruption after the person has returned home. Many families can cope with residual physical problems but find such subtle personality changes very difficult to manage.

Such changes are difficult to ameliorate and there is often little that can be done except offer counselling or psychotherapy to support the family. Sometimes a behavioural programme can improve the situation, particularly with regard to irritability or aggression. It is often surprisingly difficult to help the problems of reduced drive and lack of initiative.

Clinical depression or clinical anxiety are also quite common at some point during the recovery phase and are said to occur in around 50% of both head-injured people and carers. These problems often occur soon after return home and once again this emphasizes the need for support at this time. Occasionally profound psychiatric problems can emerge such as psychosis, mania, or obsessive compulsive disorder either in a previously predisposed individual or perhaps as a result of direct organic brain damage. The involvement of a neuropsychiatrist is important in such cases. Depression and anxiety also need active and sometimes aggressive treatment.

Later-stage rehabilitation

The previous sections have emphasized the importance of long-term community-based support. Discharge from the rehabilitation centre will often occur after a few months and there can be many months of further natural recovery requiring an active rehabilitation programme. Even if natural recovery has ceased then there is still a need for support to avoid the emergence of unnecessary physical, cognitive, intellectual, behavioural, and emotional complications.

Independent living skills and social skills

There is emerging evidence of the efficacy of specific training programmes for independent living skills, such as cooking, shopping, and community mobility. There are now a number of separate 'transitional living units' that specialize in this area. They are often funded from medico-legal assessments and there are a few available on the National Health Service. Such units will also teach a wide range of social skills, such as skills at initiating and carrying on a conversation, retaining friends, finding appropriate social outlets, interests and hobbies, etc.

Vocational rehabilitation

Regrettably it is common for brain-injured people not to return to work, or if they do return to work then lose their job because of the whole range of cognitive, behavioural, and emotional problems that often develop. There is evidence from the USA that a 'job coach' system improves the chance of finding and retaining work. The job coach is a skilled vocational counsellor who will work with the brain-injured person and slowly reintroduce them to the work environment. They will work alongside the person on the job helping them to adapt not only to the work itself but to the necessary social and interpersonal skills that go with the job. This will help to educate and train colleagues as well as more senior managers and employers. One study doubled the employment rate after the introduction of such a scheme. There are a few vocational rehabilitation units in the UK but mainly in the private sector and once again funded out of damages from a legal settlement.

Case management

In the later stages the involvement of a wide range of health, social service, and employment professionals is often needed. Access and coordination of these different professionals can be a major problem for the disabled person and their family. It is becoming increasingly common for a case manager to be appointed who can assist with such coordination and who can often act as an advocate for the disabled person and their family. For some contact need only be in the short term, but in many people after severe brain injury life-long support is needed from the case manager and many members of the rehabilitation team.

References

1 Teasdale, G. and Jennett, B. (1974). Assessment of coma and impaired consciousness. A practical scale. *Lancet* **2**: 81–3.

2 Teasdale, G., Knill-Jones, R., and Van der Sande, J. (1978). Observer variability in assessing impaired consciousness and coma. *Journal of Neurology, Neurosurgery and Psychiatry* **41**: 603–10.

3 Teasdale, G., Murray, G., Parker, L., and Jennett, B. (1979). Adding up the Glasgow Coma Scale. *Acta Neurochirurgica* **28**(Suppl.): 13–16.

Spinal cord injury

Background

Spinal cord injury is an excellent example of the improvement in survival and quality of life that can follow from a modern rehabilitation programme. In the early part of the twentieth century nine out of ten people with spinal cord injury died within 1 year and only 1% survived in the long term. Now life expectancy is only modestly reduced. A 20-year-old male would normally be expected to have around 58 years of further life and this is reduced to about 48 years in those with paraplegia and in those with tetraplegia to around 35 years of further life.

- Annual incidence of spinal cord injury is around 10–15 cases per million per annum.
- Mean age of injury is 33 years and the mode 19 years.
- Most injuries occur in males (around 82%).
- The commonest cause is road traffic accidents (40%) but with an increasing proportion from violence and a significant proportion from domestic and industrial falls and sporting injuries.

The incidence of road traffic injuries is reducing secondary to seat-belt legislation, traffic calming measures, and car safety devices.

Early acute management

At the roadside it is important to avoid unnecessary worsening of the spinal cord injury. Individuals should be immobilized in a semi-rigid collar and the individual, if other injuries allow, should be placed in a lateral position with the head kept in line with the spine by the underlying arm. Transportation should be on a spinal board with the head immobilized. Speed of evacuation is important and individuals should be transferred as soon as possible to a regional spinal injuries unit (other life-threatening injuries may need treatment before transfer).

The level of spinal injury cannot be determined solely by examination. There may be some bruising, tenderness, or deformity but there may be no clue as to the exact nature and extent of the underlying injury. Radiographic and MRI scanning is often necessary.

Initial management of injuries to the cervical spine would usually consist of skeletal traction applied through skull callipers. This will help stabilize and splint the spine. The standard initial treatment for thoracic and lumbar injuries is simple support in the correct posture usually with a pillow under the lumbar spine to maintain the normal lordosis.

It is very controversial whether conservative management is sufficient or whether operative fixation of the damaged spine produces better results. Around 60% of people in the United States undergo spinal surgery but the incidence in the UK and other parts of Western Europe is much lower. In the UK surgical intervention is reserved for those with unstable displaced fractures and conservative management is the normal practice for stable and undisplaced fractures.

Some centres use a short course of high-dose methylprednisolone in the early stages, started within at least 8 h of injury. This may improve eventual outcome.

Dermatomes, myotomes, and associated reflexes

These are summarized in Fig. 20.1.

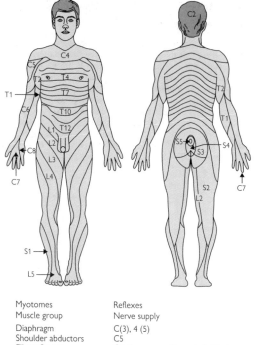

Myotomes	Reflexes	
Muscle group	Nerve supply	
Diaphragm	C(3), 4 (5)	
Shoulder abductors	C5	
Elbow flexors	C5, 6	Biceps jerk C5, 6
Supinators/pronators	C6	Supinator jerk C6
Wrist extensors	C6	
Wrist flexors	C7	
Elbow extensors	C7	Triceps jerk C7
Finger extensors	C7	
Finger flexors	C8	
Intrinisc hard muscles	T1	Abdominal reflex T8-12
Hip flexors	L1, 2	
Hip adductors	L2, 3	
Knee extensors	L3, 4	Knee jerk L3, 4
Anide dorsiflexors	L4, 5	
Toe extensors	L5	
Knee flexors	L4, 5 S1	
Ankle plantar flexors	S1,2	Ankle jerk S1, 2
Toe flexors	S1,2	
Anal sphincter	S2, 3, 4	Bulbocavernosus reflex S3, 4
		Anal reflex S5
		Plantar reflex

Fig. 20.1 An *aide mémoire* to examination—summary of the dermatomes, myotomes, and associated reflexes.

General post-acute management: management of the spine

Most people will be managed conservatively. However, one advantage of considering surgery is that the individual can be mobilized more quickly. If a conservative approach is adopted mobilization is more difficult in the first few weeks. Cervical spine traction is usually maintained for around 6 weeks and at this point individuals must be carefully monitored to make sure there are no respiratory problems and pressure sores are avoided. Once the fracture site is stable the individual can be sat up in bed and normally a halo brace can be used instead of skull traction. This allows early mobilization. The halo brace is kept on for 10–12 weeks until the site is properly stable. In thoraco-lumbar injuries the period of bed rest will usually be 8–12 weeks followed by bracing and gradual mobilization.

General post-acute management: management of medical problems

In the early stages careful monitoring needs to take place to avoid unnecessary medical complications. These mainly consist of:

Respiratory problems

Respiratory insufficiency can occur in people with cervical cord injuries as the intercostal muscles can be paralysed and in high cervical lesions the diaphragm can also be paralysed. Respiratory function can decline quite quickly and careful monitoring needs to be maintained. Regular chest physiotherapy is vital. Pulmonary embolism is also a risk and anti-coagulation is usually advised.

Pressure sores

There is a high risk of pressure sores. Individuals will need to be nursed on a pressure-relieving mattress and their position regularly changed. The skin must be kept clean. Pressure sores are nearly always preventable. If they occur they can be very slow to heal and sometimes plastic surgery is required. Septicaemia from pressure sores is still one of the leading causes of death in people with spinal injury.

Bladder problems

In the period of spinal shock the bladder is usually non-contractile so that catheterization may be appropriate. Once spinal shock has worn off the commonest problem is detrusor hyper-reflexia giving rise to frequent passage of small quantities of urine associated with urgency. Detrusor sphincter dyssynergia and detrusor hypo-reflexia are also possible, the latter tending to occur when there is damage to the sacral nerves. The management of bladder difficulties is outlined in Chapter 7.

Bowel care

In the period of spinal shock the bowel remains flaccid and should not be allowed to over-distend. Manual evacuation is usually needed. Later bowel evacuation can usually be triggered by glycerine suppository or by anal digital stimulation. Advice on a good-quality high-fibre diet is necessary in the longer term.

Spasticity and contractures

Spasticity can be a major problem in spinal injury. Contractures are nearly always preventable by careful positioning, physiotherapy, and anti-spastic treatment, such as botulinum toxin. The management of spasticity is covered in further detail in Chapter 6.

Heterotopic ossification

This is the development of bone in an abnormal anatomical position in the soft tissues. It is reasonably common in spinal cord injuries, although the prevalence varies between 5% and 50%. It commonly occurs around hips and knees, causing a decrease in range of movement and sometimes localized swelling, joint effusion, and pain. Treatment is difficult. Etidromate disodium

(Didronel) is probably the most useful treatment. Surgical intervention is usually unsatisfactory.

Deep venous thrombosis

This is a significant problem after spinal injury. Heparin is generally used as a prophylactic but some centres now also use external pneumatic calf compression.

Pain and dysaesthesia

Peripheral pain is quite common. Deep burning neuralgic pain can also occur. This is often resistant to treatment but can respond to the use of anti-convulsants and tricyclic anti-depressants. Pain from other sources, such as musculoskeletal causes and osteoarthritis, can also occur.

Autonomic dysreflexia

This is a potentially fatal problem seen in cervical cord injuries above the sympathetic outflow but sometimes in those with high thoracic lesions above T6. It is categorized by:

- Exaggerated autonomic response to a stimulus below the level of the lesion. Such stimuli can include:
  - Distension of the pelvic organs, such as bladder, colon, and rectum.
  - Catheterization.
  - Urinary infections.
  - Sexual intercourse.
  - Pressure sores.
  - Tight clothing.
  - Surgical procedures.
- Symptoms consist of:
  - Headaches.
  - Sweating.
  - Vasodilatation.
  - Nasal obstruction.
  - Paraesthesia.
  - Anxiety.
  - Significant hypertension.

Awareness of the problem is important and avoidance of unnecessary stimulation is clearly desirable. Treatment is directed towards reducing blood pressure. Sublingual nifedipine or intravenous hydralazine can be used in more severe cases. Chlorpromazine is another possibility.

Later rehabilitation

Once the individual is mobilizing then rehabilitation can continue at a greater pace. At the point of mobilization it should have become clearer about final functional level of the spinal injury. Initial recovery may have taken place and an accurate functional assessment can be carried out. The level of the lesion clearly has an important bearing on functional outcome (Table 20.1).

Table 20.1 Expected residual functional ability according to the level of lesion

Level of injury	Complete lesions
Lesion below C3	Dependent on others for all care
	Diaphragm paralysed, needs permanent ventilation or diaphragm pacing
	Chin-, head-, or breath-controlled electric wheelchair
Lesion below C4	Dependent on others for all care
	Can breathe independently using diaphragm
	Can shrug shoulders
	Can use electric wheelchair with chin control
	Can type/use computer with a mouth stick
	Environmental control system operated by shoulder shrug or mouthpiece
Lesion below C5	Can move shoulders and flex elbows
	Can eat with a feeding strap/universal cuff
	Can wash face, comb hair, clean teeth using feeding strap/universal cuff
	Can write using individually designed splint and wrist support
	Can help in dressing upper half of body
	Can push manual wheelchair short distances on the flat provided that pushing gloves are used with capstan rims on the wheels
	May be able to transfer across level surfaces using sliding board and a helper
	Electric wheelchair needed for functional mobility
Lesion below C6	Can extend wrists
	Still needs strap to eat and for self-care
	Can write using individually designed splint but may not need wrist support
	Can dress upper half of body unaided
	Can help in dressing lower half of body
	Can propel wheelchair up gentle slopes
	Can be independent in bed, car, and toilet transfers
	Can drive with hand controls
Lesion below C7	Full wrist movement and some hand function, but no finger flexion or fine hand movements
	Can do all transfers, eat, and dress independently
	Can drive with hand controls
Lesion below C8	All hand muscles except intrinsics preserved
	Wheelchair independent, but difficulty in going up and down kerbs
	Can drive with hand controls
Lesion below T1	Complete innervation of arms
	Totally independent wheelchair life
	Can drive with hand controls

Longer-term issues

Discharge home

This is a particularly difficult time. It is better to have a phased discharge with trial home visits. Very commonly houses will need adaptation for a wheelchair and other structural alternations made to improve access, both internal and external. Sometimes hoisting equipment will need to be put into the house and adaptations made to the toilet, bathroom, and kitchen. Environmental control equipment may be needed. There is a need for psychological support over this period of transition both for the injured person and their family. Anxiety and depression are both common at this time. There needs to be smooth transition and a case conference between hospital and community staff is an absolute requirement. Contact with the spinal unit should be maintained and many centres now have outreach workers who can monitor the situation and refer the individual back to the specialist care in the centre as necessary.

Emotional problems

This can be a very anxious time for the injured person as well as family and friends. Clinical depression is common and occurs at some point in at least 50% of spinal-injured people. There is some risk of suicide. Counselling and psychological support is vital and sometimes medication is needed.

Sexual life

Sexual ability depends on the level and completeness of the spinal lesion. People with complete upper motor neuron lesions will have reflex but not psychogenic erections. Even reflex erections are usually impossible in those with parasympathetic lesions. Satisfactory erection can often be achieved by mechanical means, such as vacuum erection or compressive retainer rings or intracavernosal drugs. However, the introduction of sildenafil (Viagra) is now reducing the need for such mechanical assistance. Orgasm remains possible even in those with complete spinal cord lesions. In women problems can result from lack of vaginal lubrication. Self-image and self-confidence can be severely affected and sexual counselling is often required. Individuals should be counselled about the totality of sexuality as there is a tendency for discussions to focus on penetrative sexual intercourse.

Fertility

Fertility is usually not reduced in women. However, fertility is often reduced in men who have low sperm counts with diminished sperm motility. Sometimes if ejaculation is not possible it can be induced by direct stimulation or by electroejaculation. Fertility can be improved by techniques such as *in vitro* fertilization or intracytoplasmic sperm injection. Women with spinal cord injury may have problems in labour, particularly if the lesion is above T10 and autonomic dysreflexia is a risk. However, this should not necessarily discourage women from becoming pregnant as good quality obstetric care will clearly reduce such risks.

Later medical complications

Pathological fractures
As there is a higher risk of osteoporosis in paralysed limbs then there is an increased risk of pathological fractures.

Post-traumatic syringomyelia
This occurs in about 4% of people and consists of an ascending myelopathy due to secondary cavitation in the central part of the cord. It usually presents with pain in the arm with characteristic disassociated sensory loss—reduced pain and temperature sensation but preservation of proprioception. Motor loss of the lower motor neuron type occurs and a sensory loss can spread to the face (syringobulbia). Surgical treatment includes decompression and drainage of the central cavity.

Respiratory management
Those with high cervical cord lesions who have lost diaphragmatic function require long-term ventilatory support. Modern ventilators can be mounted on a wheelchair. Speech is possible with an uncuffed tracheostomy tube that allows air to escape to the larynx and in some people a phrenic nerve stimulator can achieve diaphragmatic ventilation.

Issues of participation

Leisure pursuits

There are now a wide variety of leisure pursuits possible for those with spinal cord injury. Ideally integration to able-bodied clubs should be encouraged but there are specific clubs for those with spinal injuries, particularly wheelchair sports.

Driving

Driving a motor vehicle in modern society is increasingly vital. Driving should be possible at all levels of spinal injury except perhaps for those with very high cervical cord lesions. Automatic transmission is important and hand controls are usually essential. A variety of infra-red devices to control secondary function, such as windscreen wipers, lights, and horn are available. Very light powered steering makes life easier for those with a weak grip. Individuals with cervical lesions who retain some useful shoulder and upper function can still drive a car using a variety of driving devices attached to the steering wheel. There are a number of devices that can stow a wheelchair safely. Adapted vehicles are now readily available, if expensive, to enable people to drive from their wheelchair. The UK now has a number of specialist driving assessment centres for proper assessment of the necessary adaptations.

Employment

Regrettably only around 25–35% of people with spinal cord injuries return to work. The chances are higher in younger people or those already in a job at the time of injury. Although returning to and retaining a job is not easy individuals should be encouraged to contact the disablement employment advisors who can provide both advice and financial help.

Information

The key to independence is access to good quality information. Individuals should be kept informed of developments at all times and put in touch with the necessary range of professionals, not only health but also in social services, employment, and in other spheres. Much valuable support can be gained from the local spinal injuries association. The internet now provides an excellent source of information and advice and training in computer literacy should be encouraged by the rehabilitation team.

The management of spinal cord injury can pose a range of challenges to the multidisciplinary team. At the present time we cannot yet promote natural recovery but many useful interventions are possible. Individuals with spinal injury can certainly continue to have a good quality of life and many should be able to work and fully participate in society.

Parkinson's disease and movement disorders

Parkinson's disease

In the last 30 years there have been huge improvements in the drug therapy of Parkinson's disease so that in the early stages disability and handicap are kept to a minimum. However, in the later stages there is a less satisfactory response to dopaminergic therapy and major problems of disability and handicap can arise. Thus, Parkinson's disease is still a major rehabilitation challenge, often to the geriatric rehabilitation team.

Causes of Parkinsonism

It is important to remember that there are many different causes of Parkinsonism some of which need specific treatment in their own right (e.g. Wilson's disease). Table 21.1 outlines some of the causes of Parkinsonism.

The importance of awareness of the different causes of Parkinsonism is not only that some need different treatments but that others respond much less well to standard dopaminergic therapy. Progressive supra-nuclear palsy and various multiple system atrophies, for example, do not respond at all well to therapeutic intervention and symptom management becomes the mainstay of rehabilitation.

Epidemiology

Parkinson's disease is by the far most common cause of Parkinsonism. The prevalence is around 150–200 per 100 000 population in the UK and an incidence of 18–20 per 100 000 population per annum. The male/female ratio is around 3:2. The disorder becomes much more common with increasing age, and approximately 1 in 10 people over the age of 80 will have Parkinsonism of various causes. However, the mean age of onset is 55 years and so it is not exclusively a problem of the older population and can occur in people who are still economically active.

Table 21.1 Causes of Parkinsonism

Class of disorder	Manifestation
Degenerative diseases	Parkinson's disease
	Progressive supra nuclear palsy
	Multiple system atrophies
	Olivopontocerebellar atrophy
Infections	Post encephalitic Parkinsonism
Drug or toxin induced	Neuroleptics
	Carbon monoxide poisoning
	Manganese poisoning
	MPTP-induced Parkinsonism
Vascular conditions	Cerebrovascular disease
	Hypertensive encephalopathy
Trauma	Head injury
	Punch drunk syndrome
Cerebral tumour	Alzheimer's disease
Other neurological conditions that may have Parkinsonian features	Intermittently raised pressure hydrocephalus
	Various forms of Huntington's disease
	Wilson's disease

MPTP, methyl-4-phenyl-1,2,3,6-tetrahydropyridine.

Principal features

There are three main features of Parkinson's disease:

- Hypokinesis or reduced movement, including
  - delay in initiation
  - poverty of movement
  - imprecision
  - slowness of movement (bradykinesia)
  - fatigue
  - problems with automatically associated movements (such as arm swing and reduction of facial expression).
- Rigidity:
  - Increased resistance to passive muscle stretch throughout the range of movement (lead pipe).
  - Rigidity is usually present in the trunk as well as the limb muscles.
  - Rigidity is responsible for the stooped posture characteristic of the disease.
- Tremor:
  - Is usually a slow coarse rest tremor and is often more of an embarrassment than a functional problem.
  - It is usually the hypokinesis and rigidity that cause the main functional difficulties.

The other component is *impaired postural reflexes*. The individual pushed from in front tends to stagger backwards or pushed from behind tend to stumble forwards. This disequilibrium is often reflected in everyday difficulties such as maintaining balance in a crowded environment or when trying to hurry or change direction.

Medical management

The details of medical management are the subject of neurological text-books. However, as the medical management is the mainstay of treatment in Parkinson's disease some relevant points can be made.

The key to treatment of Parkinson's disease is direct replacement of levodopa which needs to be combined with carbidopa (a peripheral decar-boxylase inhibitor) that reduces peripheral side-effects. There are now many combinations of carbidopa/levodopa as well as various controlled-release forms. Drugs come in different formats, such as tablets or liquids. It is often a matter of trial and error to find the right balance of appro-priate dopa replacement therapy. In general terms it is usually best to give smaller doses at frequent intervals throughout the day. Obviously the minimum dose compatible with the desired reduction in symptom levels is necessary. This should mean that treatment varies according to the handi-cap of the individual. Treatment is usually more aggressive in a younger person who is still at work and needs a reasonable degree of control and coordination—sometimes at the expense of side-effects. In the older person who simply needs to get around the house adequately then a less aggressive treatment is necessary. In the older person side-effects are usually more problematic.

Some authorities would start treatment as soon as the diagnosis is made, while others would wait as late as possible so that the complica-tions of treatment are delayed. There is still no clear consensus on this issue. However, most people would now start treatment as and when symptoms become troublesome and interfere with daily life. Once again this usually means early intervention for the young active person and later intervention for disabled elderly people. The general treatments now available are:

- Dopa replacement therapy—Sinemet or Madopar in various formats.
- Dopamine agonist agents, such as bromocriptine, pergolide, lysuride, cabergoline, or ropinirole.
- Dopamine B-oxidase inhibitors—selegiline, thought to slow progression of disease until more recent studies have thrown some doubts on long-term efficacy and safety.
- Anticholinergic drugs can be useful in milder cases although troublesome side-effects include confusion, dry mouth, blurred vision, constipation, and impaired erection.
- Self-injected apomorphine (direct acting D_1 dopamine agonist with rapid onset of action) can be useful when there are late-stage complications and 'rescue' is required from a bad rigid period.

Any form of dopamine replacement therapy is usually very effective for several years. However, after 5–10 years of treatment difficulties can begin to arise. The person can begin to swing from a rigid phase ('off') to a phase of marked dyskinetic movements ('on'). This on/off swinging can be manifest in a variety of patterns, and the dosage and timing of treatment becomes increasingly difficult. At this point the input of a specialist neuro-logical Parkinson's disease service becomes necessary.

There has recently been renewed interest in stereotactic neurosurgical procedures, usually deep stimulation of three target areas—the thalamus, subthalamic nucleus, and globus pallidus. There has also been recent interest in implantation or neural grafting techniques to boost cerebral dopamine production but such techniques are neither widely proven nor widely available.

Rating scales

Accurate clinical assessment is a fundamental part of rehabilitation medicine and assessment in Parkinson's disease is no exception. As usual, individual symptoms should have their own measures but it is sometimes useful to have an overall disability rating scale. There are a few that have been validated for Parkinson's disease. The commonest are the staging scales of Hoehn and Yahr and the disease rating scales of Webster (Tables 21.2 and 21.3). There are other more comprehensive tools, such as the Unified Parkinson's Disease Rating Scale, that are mainly used for research purposes.

Table 21.2 Standard scales in Parkinson's disease: staging (Hoehn and Yahr 1967)

Stage	Description
I	Unilateral involvement, little or no functional impairment
II	Bilateral or midline involvement without impaired balance
III	First signs of impaired writing reflexes; some functional restriction but capable of independent living and may be able to work
IV	Fully developed severe disabling disease; can stand and walk unaided
V	Confined to wheelchair or bed

(After Hoehn, M.M., Yahr, M.D. (1967). Parkinsonism: onset, progression and mortality. *Neurology* **17**: 427–42.

Table 21.3 Standard scales in Parkinson's disease: disease rating (Webster 1968). A clinical rating (0–3) is given for each of the 10 items with 0 = no involvement and 3 = severe (instructions being given for each)

Item	
1	Bradykinesia of hands (including handwriting and pronation–supination)
2	Rigidity: proximal and distal
3	Posture: head flexion, 'poker' spine, and simian posture
4	Upper extremity swing
5	Gait: stride length, shuffling
6	Tremor: amplitude and constancy
7	Facies: mobility
8	Seborrhoea
9	Speech
10	Self-care

(After Webster, D.D. (1968). Critical analysis of the disability in Parkinson's disease. *Mod Treat.* **5**:257–82.

Treatment of symptoms in Parkinson's disease

Gait

The most obvious problem in Parkinson's disease is the shuffling and unsafe gait which can cause frequent falls. Bradykinesia and rigidity are the problems largely responsible, combined with impaired postural reflexes. The gait problems can also be made worse by dyskinetic movements as a result of treatment.

There is now evidence that a physiotherapist can definitely improve gait, although the exact type and duration of therapy is not really known. It is probable that a home-based physiotherapy programme is useful and is certainly the most appreciated by the individual.

The physiotherapist can teach various trick strategies that can overcome some of the problems. Some examples are:

- Freezing—in this phenomenon the individual suddenly freezes as if the feet were stuck to the floor. This can be helped by getting the person to pretend that they have to step over a small obstruction. Freezing in a chair can be helped by being taught to gently rock backwards and forwards until there is sufficient momentum to rise.
- The slow and shuffling gait can be improved by auditory cues.
- Severe and painful rigidity can be helped by simple stretching exercises.
- There seems to be some value (probably psychological and social as well as physical) in group therapy sessions.

It is important that physiotherapy contact is maintained throughout the illness. Short bursts of physiotherapy for further training and advice is probably the best methodology available when there are scarce resources. The physiotherapist will often have to work in conjunction with the neurologist or geriatrician so that the drug therapy can be manipulated in order to maximize mobility at the most relevant times of day for that individual.

Activities of daily living

The same problems of bradykinesia, rigidity, and tremor will often cause problems with fine hand and arm movements. Involvement by the occupational therapist and other team members can make real improvements. There is now a large variety of suitable aids that can assist including:

- Large-handled cutlery.
- Plate guards.
- Use of Velcro instead of buttons.
- Writing aids.
- Various home-based assessments in order to maximize functional use in the kitchen, bedroom, bathroom, etc.

Speech and swallowing problems

Communication can become difficult in Parkinsonism. The speech is characteristically described as dysarthrophonic—a combination of problems of articulation and phonation. It is usually a monotonous pitch combined with a quiet voice with words coming in short rushes at variable rates due to the impaired breath control. Stuttering can also occur. Referral to a speech therapist is useful at the earliest possible stage. Appropriate speech exercises can produce significant improvements in intonation, stress, and rhythm and in more advanced stages various forms of augmentative communication aid can be prescribed.

Regrettably the problem of coordination also affects swallowing. The assessment of swallowing is described in Chapter 9. The involvement of a speech therapist, dietician, and radiographer is essential. Dietary manipulation may be needed, and accurate diagnosis rests on videofluroscopy. There are various speech techniques that can improve swallowing, although most emphasis is usually placed on appropriate changes in food consistency whilst maintaining adequate nutritional intake.

Autonomic problems

Problems with bladder function occur in around 50% of people with Parkinson's disease and are probably secondary to autonomic dysfunction which occurs as part of the disease process. The commonest symptoms are:

- Frequency.
- Urgency.
- Urge incontinence.
- Sometimes hesitancy and retention.

The situation can be complicated and urodynamic evaluation is often necessary. Other problems of autonomic function can also occur. The commonest is *postural hypotension* often leading to fainting on getting out of bed or getting up from a seat. This occurs more commonly in some of the other Parkinsonian syndromes, particularly the Shy–Drager syndrome and other Parkinson plus syndromes. Treatment is difficult but can include:

- Advice on avoiding rapid changes of posture.
- Avoiding large meals.
- Avoiding excessive alcohol.
- Avoiding warm temperatures.
- Avoiding excessive straining.
- Use of compressive garments, such as elastic stockings or abdominal binders (often impractical).
- Treatment with fludrocortisone.

Constipation is also common, although drugs, particularly anticholinergic drugs, might be responsible. Dietary manipulation can be helpful as well as adopting a regular pattern of defecation. Laxatives and other bulk forming agents should be avoided if at all possible but can be helpful in resistant cases.

Pain

It is usually thought that sensory symptoms are not present in Parkinson's disease and sensory signs are absent. However, it is quite common for cramp-like pains and diffuse aches and pains to be present. In an older population such difficulties can of course be secondary to musculoskeletal problems, such as a result of osteoarthritis. Sometimes pain can go hand in hand with the short-term disease fluctuations, such as the on/off swinging, which can be helped by appropriate drug manipulation.

Treatment of symptoms in Parkinson's disease (*continued*)

Sleep disorders

Disorders of sleep are very common in Parkinson's disease. The commonest is sleep fragmentation characterized by recurrent waking which may in turn be due to the inability to turn over at night because of the bradykinesia and rigidity. Daytime fatigue is consequently common. Drug manipulation might be needed in order to try to get an appropriate dopaminergic effect overnight. There are now various devices that can help someone turn over in bed. These vary from the very simple, such as a strap attached to the bed head, or the even simpler device of wearing cotton socks which gives some purchase on the sheets. There are now also automatic beds that will tip slightly helping the individual turn over.

Sexual function

It is likely that the autonomic dysfunction in Parkinson's disease can also result in problems of erection in the male. In addition both sexes can be troubled by mechanical problems during sex secondary to the physical impairments. The situation is often compounded by drug effects, particularly anticholinergics which can dry secretions and cause erectile problems. The involvement of a sexual counsellor is useful. Sexual problems can often be helped by:

- Simple advice on timing of drugs.
- Advice on posture.
- Counselling to deal with problems of self-image and relationship difficulties.
- Alternative means of sexual stimulation.

Cognitive and emotional problems

Depression is very common in Parkinson's disease and occurs in over 50% of the Parkinsonian population at some point during the disease. As in many neurological problems there is a tendency to assume that depression is a natural accompaniment of the disorder and for it not to be treated adequately. There is no evidence that depression in the context of Parkinson's disease responds any worse than depression in other contexts and it should be treated just as aggressively (see Chapter 14).

Clinical anxiety can also be a problem but is normally a result of inadequate information, advice, and counselling.

Dementia is undoubtedly more common in Parkinson's disease and the incidence is around 20–30%. It is obviously more common in other forms of Parkinsonism and indeed Parkinsonism can be associated with Alzheimer's disease itself. Dementia in the context of Parkinson's disease is often characterized by:

- Increasing dependency.
- Increasing indecision.
- Increasing passivity.
- Memory problems.
- Perseveration.

- Slowness of thought.
- Problems with new learning.
- Increasing 'mental' inflexibility.

It is often the dementia that causes increasing family stress and involvement of psychogeriatric services can be needed in the later stages.

Issues in service delivery

The preceding sections have shown that there is a wide range of problems in Parkinson's disease requiring input from a whole multidisciplinary team. In the case of Parkinson's disease the team should undoubtedly have medical input, usually from a neurologist or geriatrician with a particular interest in Parkinson's. There are now a number of hospital or community-based Parkinson's teams providing long-term contact, help, and advice. As with all chronic neurological problems, accurate information, advice, and counselling, not only to the affected person but also to the family, is vital at all stages.

Individuals should be put in contact with local Parkinson's disease or other relevant societies, which can provide useful literature written in lay terms.

Fortunately in the UK there has been the development of specialist nurses specifically trained in the management of Parkinson's disease. Such nurse practitioners can provide invaluable help, advice, and support, including advice on drug manipulation. This reduces the amount of time the individual may need to spend in neurological or geriatric outpatient clinics. The nurse practitioner could be the main point of contact for access to the whole variety of health and social services.

Dystonia

Dystonia is defined as a sustained involuntary muscle contraction involving abnormal movements and postures. There are many types of presentation and some of the commoner sites are as follows:

- Neck—spasmodic torticollis or cervical dystonia.
- Eye—blepharospasm.
- Jaw, tongue, and mouth—oromandibular dystonia.
- Larynx and vocal cords—spasmodic dysphonia.
- Arm and hand muscles—various segmental, multifocal, and hemidystonic forms.
- Generalized dystonia—usually but not invariably starting in childhood.

In addition there are various occupational cramps which usually, but not always, occur in the context of an occupation with repetitive movements, such as writer's cramp or various musician's cramps or sportsman cramps, such as dystonia of the hand muscles occurring in professional darts players.

The dystonias are uncommon but not rare. A recent survey showed a prevalence of around 26 per 100 000 population for all types of dystonia.

Aetiology is normally unknown, although there is emerging evidence of a genetic predisposition and now at least 20 genetic disorders are described in specific dystonic families. It is likely that dystonia has a genetic predisposition but requires an environmental trigger—which is usually unknown. Occasionally dystonia can be symptomatic of another process and a thorough neurological examination and, if necessary, investigation is needed. Hemidystonia, for example, can follow stroke or traumatic brain injury or be a manifestation of underlying brain tumour.

Important secondary causes are drug-induced dystonias, caused by the psychotrophic medications for example.

Treatment

In a few cases specific treatment is required, such as in Wilson's disease. Occasionally surgical removal of tumours or arterior venous malformations might be needed. However, in the vast majority of cases such specific measures are not possible. The treatment of choice for the focal dystonias is now undoubtedly *botulinum toxin*. Botulinum toxin acts by blocking the transmission of acetylcholine at nerve endings and thus weakening the appropriate muscles. The toxin is delivered by intramuscular injection and takes two to three days to take effect. The effect then lasts around 3 months before new nerve endings sprout and the injection needs repeating. The injection is remarkably safe and the only real problem is a flu-like illness occurring in about 1% of those injected. Sometimes there can be difficulties of over-weakening the injected muscles, such as dysphagia as a complication of injection for spasmodic torticollis.

In a few people (around 5–10%) the injection does not work or there is later non-response probably due to the formation of antibodies. In such cases the use of oral drug therapy may still be necessary.

The prescription of the right drug can be time-consuming. Overall around 40% of people find a drug that suits their dystonia but about half of these individuals have unacceptable side-effects. Thus, only about one in

five people will eventually find a drug that is appropriate and helpful. The drugs that can be used are:
- Anticholinergics.
- Muscle relaxants—baclofen.
- Benzodiazepines such as clonazepam.
- Dopamine agonists (there is a rare form of dystonia that responds immediately and extremely well to dopamine but the other forms of dystonia can sometimes respond reasonably well).
- Dopamine antagonists.

Sometimes surgical procedures can be useful. There are various procedures for specific focal dystonias. These include:
- Surgery to lift the eyelids in blepharospasm.
- Surgery on the neck muscles for spasmodic torticollis.
- Various forms of brain ablative or stimulation procedures, particularly for hemidystonias.

Other therapy

As dystonia is such an unusual condition it is important that good-quality literature is given for information, help, and advice. The Dystonia Society produces excellent and readable literature in the UK. Depression and anxiety can occur and access to a counsellor can be helpful. There is some evidence that complementary medicine, such as hypnotherapy and acupuncture, can help in certain resistant cases. Various members of the multidisciplinary team may need to be called upon for advice, such as the speech therapist for dysphonia, or the full team may be needed for the more widespread generalized dystonias.

Huntington's disease

Huntington's disease is a rare condition with a prevalence of only around 2–10 per 100 000 population. It is a degenerative disorder in which neuronal loss occurs in the caudate nucleus and putamen with a characteristic finding of atrophy in the head of the caudate nucleus on MRI scanning.

Genetics

Huntington's disease is an autosomal dominant condition with virtually full penetrance so that each offspring of an affected parent has a one in two risk of inheriting the disorder. The gene has now been mapped (to the tip of the short arm of chromosome 4) and the responsible gene was identified in 1993. A diagnostic test is now available with a very high sensitivity and specificity—virtually 100%. Genetic counselling is key to management in this disorder as pre-symptomatic testing is now possible. There are now useful protocols for the management of pre-symptomatic testing and such testing should be carried out only in recognized centres. The protocol typically includes:

- One or two sessions on the general features and inheritance of Huntington's disease.
- The next few sessions concentrate on the issues of pre-symptomatic testing and a blood sample is taken if the client wishes to go ahead.
- One pre-test session is initially arranged with a psychiatrist to reduce the risk of severe psychiatric reaction following the test.
- A session where the result is given on a face to face basis.
- Appropriate follow-up arrangements, particularly counselling, both after a positive result and after a negative result. Contact should be made soon after the result either by telephone or a home visit.

The peak age of onset is around 40 years, which obviously means that the person is often married with a young family and thus with a high risk of having passed on the genetic defect to the offspring. Onset can rarely occur before the age of 20 and rarely after 60. Onset is insidious but time from diagnosis to death is around 10–15 years. There is a characteristic spectrum of motor, psychiatric, and cognitive problems.

Motor features

Involuntary movements, particularly chorea, are seen in most, but not all, people. Facial chorea is particularly common. Gait can be unsteady and dyspraxic. Dysarthria can occur and swallowing can be compromised. Sometimes other involuntary movements are present, such as dystonia. Apraxia can also occur when testing the arm.

Psychiatric disorders

Psychiatric problems are virtually universal. Often there are insidious changes in personality and behaviour that pre-date the first physical symptoms. Apathy can be present but a more common pattern is irritability with outbursts of verbal and physical aggression. Sometimes an individual will go on to more overt psychiatric illness including major depression or even schizophrenia-like manifestations. Euphoria and manic episodes have also been reported.

Cognitive impairment

There is a wide range of cognitive problems even in the early stages of Huntington's disease. Subtle intellectual decline can even be detected in carriers of the genetic mutation before any symptoms are present. Speech can be halting with long pauses and there are often problems with word finding and naming difficulties. Writing can be impaired, but fortunately reading is usually reasonably well preserved. Many people report difficulty in planning, requiring considerable support and assistance from their family and carers. Visuospatial tasks can be affected, which adds to the overall dementing illness. Obviously memory problems can be particularly difficult as frank dementia progresses.

Treatment and support

Huntington's disease is not curable but a rehabilitation team can provide invaluable assistance and support:

- Physiotherapy can improve gait and reduce unnecessary physical complications, such as contractures.
- Occupational therapy can assist with activities of daily living and planning of the home and work environment.
- Speech and language therapy can be used for the management of dysphagia and communication problems.
- A dietician can be useful as there is often a significant increase in calorific requirements in someone with constant movements.
- A neuropsychological or neuropsychiatric assessment is essential as depression, behavioural problems, and dementia begin to take effect.

A dedicated team managing people with Huntington's disease in each region provides the best quality service, assistance, and support to the Huntington's population.

Chapter 22

Motor neuron diseases

Background

The motor neuron diseases usually have a progressive course leading to death within 3–5 years of diagnosis. However, there can be considerable rehabilitation potential in terms of reducing the risk of unnecessary complications and promoting quality of life. This is particularly important in motor neuron disease where people nearly always retain normal cognitive function and full conscious appreciation of their disability. It is the role of the rehabilitation team to help the individual and their family overcome the feeling of powerlessness.

Textbooks of neurology should be referred to for a detailed discussion of classification, pathology, aetiology, and diagnosis. However, there are a few points that should be mentioned which are of relevance to the rehabilitation team.

Motor neuron diseases

It is important to remember that although adult-onset motor neuron disease accounts for around 90% of cases there is an increasingly important range of other motor neuron diseases and it is very likely that over the next few years further genetic disorders will be identified which may eventually lead to different treatment possibilities. The following is an abbreviated classification of motor neuron diseases as currently understood.

- Sporadic motor neuron disease:
  - *Amyotrophic lateral sclerosis (ALS)*—mixture of upper and lower motor neuron problems giving rise to characteristic signs including spasticity, increased reflexes, and muscle weakness in combination with muscle wasting and muscle fasciculation.
  - *Progressive bulbar palsy*—a similar combination of lower and upper motor neuron problems but mainly involving the bulbar muscles giving rise to additional problems such as dribbling, dysarthria, dysphagia, and respiratory difficulties.
  - *Progressive muscular atrophy*—only affecting the lower motor neurons of the limbs with a better survival.
  - *Primary lateral sclerosis*—a rarer form only involving upper motor neurons.
- Familial motor neuron disease: accounts for around 10% of all motor neuron diseases and an increasing number (currently around 20%) have an identified genetic locus. Currently 20% have a mutation in chromosome 21 involving copper/zinc superoxide dismutase. There are other rarer genetic and inherited forms of motor neuron disease.
- Western Pacific amyotrophic lateral sclerosis/Parkinsonism/dementia complex.
- Juvenile onset motor neuron disease—with intracytoplasmic conclusions.
- Motor neuron diseases with definable causes:
  - Post-polio syndrome.
  - Heavy metal intoxication.
  - Hexosaminidase-A deficiency.

The precise diagnosis is obviously important and is likely to become increasingly important as more genetic and biochemical abnormalities are determined.

Epidemiology

The prevalence of motor neuron disease is around 5 per 100 000 population with an incidence of around 1–2 per 100 000 population per annum. There are areas of geographical concentration where the incidence exceeds 100 times the average (including the western Pacific island of Guam, several specific villages in Japan, and the Irian Jaya region of Papua New Guinea).

Motor neuron disease is mainly a disease of late middle age, with an age of onset in the 50s and 60s. There are a greater number of males than females, with a ratio of approximately 1.6:1. The average duration of symptoms to death is around 2–3 years with survival a little longer in younger patients and those with progressive muscular atrophy.

Diagnosis

The symptoms of presentation can vary enormously. Motor weakness and the absence of sensory loss is probably the most common presenting feature, although sometimes the first complaint can be of muscle cramps or fasciculations or muscle wasting. Diagnosis still rests largely on clinical history and examination often supported by neurophysiological evidence of denervation in the muscles of at least two limbs.

Giving the diagnosis

The diagnosis of motor neuron disease is usually fairly straightforward in the majority of cases. It is said that around 80% of people can be diagnosed within a few minutes, 10% need some further investigations to exclude other pathologies, and in 10% of people the diagnosis only becomes apparent after several months of symptom progression. Thus, in the majority of people an accurate diagnosis can be given quite quickly. Obviously imparting the diagnosis is a particularly anxious time for the family. The following are key points:

- Accurate information is required.
- Plenty of time is needed to impart in the diagnosis and to offer quick follow-up appointments to answer further questions.
- Counselling should be available.
- Lay literature should be given which is produced by local motor neuron disease groups or the national societies.
- It is useful to give the name and contact details of a key person such as a motor neuron disease specialist nurse or other appropriately trained individual who can answer further questions and put the person in touch with other relevant members of the rehabilitation team as and when required.
- The individual should always have access to a full range of skilled professionals, preferably in a coherent multidisciplinary rehabilitation team. If referrals are made then people need to be seen quickly and it is often appropriate to make quick loans of appropriate equipment; there are often fast track procedures for the supply of equipment to people with motor neuron disease.

Treatment and rehabilitation

Medical treatment

Regrettably, at the time of writing, there is no single agent that is confirmed to slow down disease progression. Many promising therapies have not stood the test of larger-scale double-blind, placebo-controlled studies. The most promising treatment focuses on anti-glutamate therapy and riluzole, a sodium channel blocker that inhibits glutamate release, seems to be the most promising such agent. Two large-scale studies have demonstrated a modest benefit and prolonged survival in motor neuron disease. Other large-scale studies are under way both with other anti-glutamate agents and with several neurotrophic factors. The results of these studies are still awaited.

Rehabilitation management

Mobility and activities of daily living

The combination of upper and lower motor neuron dysfunction is particularly prone to lead to weakness in combination with a risk of contractures secondary to spasticity. In the early stages advice on gait and passive exercises is important and the physiotherapist should be involved. Most people will relatively quickly progress to wheelchair dependency and then an appropriate wheelchair and seating needs to be prescribed with proper cushioning to reduce the risk of pressure sores. There is a variety of simple aids to daily living which can produce significant functional benefit and the input of both physiotherapy and occupational therapy is important for a functional assessment and treatment regime to be put into place.

Respiratory and bulbar problems

One of the most distressing difficulties arises from bulbar involvement. The following symptoms can occur:

- Dysphagia arises from muscle weakness and problems of coordination of the tongue and swallowing mechanism. An assessment by a speech and language therapist is required, often involving videofluorscopy and the involvement of a radiographer and dietician (see Chapter 9).
- Feeding can often become slow and tiring and it may be preferable to use a percutaneous endoscopic gastrostomy (PEG) feeding regime sooner rather than later. This will maintain calorific intake, reduce the length of time spent on feeding, and reduce, but not entirely remove, the risk of aspiration, pneumonia, and malnutrition.
- Dribbling can be a particular difficulty. Anti-cholinergic drugs or patches can be helpful but can be associated with troublesome side-effects, particularly constipation, dry mouth, and urinary problems. Recently, injection of the salivary glands with botulinum toxin has been shown to be useful for this troublesome symptom.
- Dysarthria and communication problems: advice from a speech and language therapist is invaluable. At the end stage short-term loan of assistive communication devices can often be helpful to maintain quality of life and the ability to communicate not only with family and friends but also strangers.
- Respiratory failure: involvement of the respiratory muscles of the neck and intercostals as well as phrenic nerve damage can all seriously compromise respiration. Physiotherapy input is important at this point

for advice and treatment regarding chest drainage, intermittent suction, and positioning. Portable suction devices should be available within the home. There may come a point when ventilatory assistance is required. At this stage ethical dilemmas are not uncommon and judgements sometimes need to be made after broad discussion with the individual, family, and the rehabilitation team as to whether quality of life would be improved in the short term by artificial ventilation or whether such measures would uncomfortably prolong life. Non-invasive intermittent positive pressure ventilation via a mask is the most practical form of assistive ventilation. The equipment is portable and can be used on a wheelchair. Ventilatory support during sleep can lead to subjective improvement in sleep and resolution of morning headaches and reduction of fatigability during the daytime. Twenty-four hour intermittent positive pressure ventilation via a tracheostomy tube is only rarely used. Antibiotics would normally be given for chest infection unless pneumonia is overwhelming. For severe anxiety or panic a small dose of lorazepam sublingually can be helpful. If breathlessness causes distress during the later stages of the disease then small amounts of morphine can be useful, even though it is a respiratory depressant.

Other features

Pain is not usually present in the early stages of motor neuron disease but is quite common in the later stages and is often due to musculoskeletal problems in combination with muscle cramps, spasticity, and other factors such as constipation. Treatment obviously depends on the cause but non-steroidal anti-inflammatory agents can be useful to ease the muscu-loskeletal aches and pains.

Emotional problems

Almost all people with motor neuron disease will go through a period of clinical anxiety and depression. Hopefully such problems need not become severe if proper support is given and counselling is available. As usual lack of knowledge goes hand in hand with unnecessary anxiety. Psychological and psychiatric support should be available as necessary. A few people have the troublesome problem of emotionalism, including pathological tearful-ness and laughter, probably because of bulbar involvement. Small doses of anti-depressants can significantly help such symptoms.

Terminal care

Most studies show that people prefer to stay at home during their terminal stage. This will often require complex, albeit short-term, care packages involving experienced nurses with the support of the rehabilitation team. Death is usually from bronchopneumonia. Small doses of morphine and/or prochlorperazine and hyoscine can be used to relieve distress and diminish bronchial secretion.

In many countries ethical questions are now arising with regard to assisted suicide. In virtually all countries this remains illegal. However, it should be pointed out that no physician has an ethical, legal, or moral obligation to prolong the distress of a dying individual. Post-bereavement counselling should also be available to the family who have often gone through a very traumatic period.

Service delivery

The preceding sections clearly demonstrate that motor neuron disease requires the complex interaction of a variety of health professionals. There is little doubt that individuals with motor neuron disease are best managed by a comprehensive multidisciplinary rehabilitation team. The team should be available to offer specialist advice at all times and regular reviews should be offered in case unrecognized complications are beginning to arise. The advent of motor neuron disease specialist nurses is a useful development, and such people can often act as the key point of contact with the rest of the team. There are now a number of examples of motor neuron disease specialist teams around the UK and abroad. Such teams often have access to a wide range of equipment and assistive technology devices, including environment control equipment and communication aids, that can be loaned in the short term.

Disorders of the peripheral nerves

Background

Accurate diagnosis is important for the rehabilitation of people with disorders of the peripheral nerves. There are a small but increasing number of disorders that are now specifically treatable. Even in those disorders of peripheral nerves that do not currently have a specific treatment accurate diagnosis remains important in order to determine natural history and prognosis. This will help to determine the rehabilitation strategy. Some conditions are spontaneously recoverable, such as Guillain–Barré syndrome, whilst others are progressive, such as the hereditary motor and sensory neuropathies. Some may require surgical intervention, such as the brachial plexus injuries. This section will cover the following disorders of peripheral nerves in order to indicate the range and extent of rehabilitation techniques:

- Critical illness polyneuropathy.
- Guillain–Barré syndrome.
- Post-polio syndrome.
- Hereditary motor and sensory neuropathies.
- Brachial plexus injuries.

Disorders of peripheral nerves usually consist, in varying proportions, of the following problems:

- Weakness—lower motor neuron weakness, particularly affecting the arms and legs.
- Variable degrees of sensory disturbance.
- Troublesome pain, either directly as a result of the peripheral nerve damage or secondary to abnormal gait and posture.
- Retained intellect.

Nerve conduction studies, *electromyography* (EMG) and sometimes *nerve biopsy* may all be necessary not only to determine the diagnosis but to determine the prognosis. There may, for example, be evidence of complete denervation (poor prognosis), partial denervation (better prognosis) or some denervation with evidence of re-innervation (good prognosis).

The following sections will deal with different types of peripheral nerve disorders from acute, severe, and reversible conditions to chronic and steadily progressive problems.

Weakness

Virtually all peripheral nerve lesions are associated with weakness, and from a functional point of view weakness affecting the arms and legs is the most disabling. In acute polyneuropathies (e.g. Guillain–Barré syndrome) weakness of the trunk muscles and respiratory muscles can clearly have a more immediate detrimental effect as respiration may be depressed. In other forms of peripheral nerve disorders there can be difficulties with swallowing or head control which brings additional rehabilitation challenges.

Weakness can cause the following problems:

- Reduced walking ability secondary to weak leg muscles.
- Easy tripping over rough ground or even carpets.
- Reduced functional ability in the arms.
- Contractures—it is usually thought that contractures are only associated with upper motor neuron spasticity but contractures of the soft tissues are not uncommon if the effects of gravity are not counteracted by appropriate splinting in individuals with lower motor neuron problems.

The following may be needed:

- Passive movements of the limbs, particularly in the acute phase, should prevent contractures.
- Splinting can restore function, particularly in the arm.
- Provision of an ankle–foot orthosis can correct weak dorsiflexion, improve gait, and prevent falls.
- Exercise can improve muscle strength, although it probably does not improve the rate of recovery of the underlying neuropathy. Isometric and isotonic exercises both increase muscle power and exercise tolerance but there is little information on the precise amount of such exercise required for maximum effect.
- People with longer-term weakness may need adaptations to their immediate environment, such as ramps, lifts, wheelchairs, special utensils, and other hand adaptations (e.g. pen holder, etc).
- Other home and work adaptations, such as environmental control equipment, can also help to reduce the disability associated with chronic arm and leg weakness.

Sensory disturbance and pain

Loss of normal sensation carries a significant risk of unnoticed trauma with the consequent dangers of *neuropathic ulceration* and *neuropathic arthropathy*. Individuals must be taught to be aware of the problem and examine areas of abnormal sensation regularly. They should be very careful with the use of appropriate footwear and expert *chiropody* is essential for those with sensory disturbance in the feet.

Involvement of sensory nerves can lead to severe *neuropathic pain*. Neuropathic pain is variously described but words often used are constant, deep, and burning. The treatment of neuropathic pain can be very difficult but may include:

• Anti-convulsants.
• Tricyclic anti-depressants.
• Cannabis or cannabinoids.
• Local or regional sympathetic blockade.
• Use of a TENS machine.

It is also important to remember that in some people an abnormal gait or posture can lead to secondary musculoskeletal pain. Involvement of a physiotherapist is vital in order to normalize gait as much as possible as well as provide appropriate seating and postural support. The most useful drugs for musculoskeletal pain are the non-steroidal anti-inflammatory agents.

Other problems can arise and will need treatment in their own right:

• Pressure sores.
• Scoliosis.
• Contractures.
• Respiratory depression (see Guillain–Barré syndrome).
• Poor nutrition, often secondary to feeding problems.
• Depression and emotional disturbance, secondary not only to the physical disability but to associated chronic pain.

Guillain–Barré syndrome and critical illness polyneuropathy

Guillain–Barré syndrome

Guillain–Barré syndrome is rare and only affects between 1–2 people per 100 000 population per year. The key features are:

- Often rapid onset usually in a matter of days but sometimes a matter of hours.
- Advancing weakness often starting in the feet but rapidly moving upwards to involve the muscles around the knees and hips and then the hands, wrists, elbows, and shoulders.
- Around 20% of people develop respiratory weakness requiring artificial ventilation.
- Can also be associated with bulbar weakness and autonomic failure.
- Treatment involves plasmapheresis and/or intravenous IgG infusion as soon as possible after the start of the illness.
- Prognosis is reasonable but a significant minority will remain disabled in the long term. A recent study showed that around 60% make a complete recovery. However, 8% die in the acute phase, 4% remain ventilator dependent, around 10% are unable to walk unaided, and the remainder have some residual physical disability.
- Prognosis is difficult to predict but older people, those unable to walk within 4 days of onset or those requiring artificial ventilation tend to have a poor outcome.
- Acute management focuses on the need to monitor respiratory function and start ventilation as necessary. Acute management will also require careful monitoring of positioning to minimize the risk of contractures and pressures.
- Urinary and chest infections are a particular risk in the early stages.
- Autonomic dysfunction can result in severe postural hypotension.
- Recovery can be slow and require a considerable amount of rehabilitation.
- Fatigue can be a real difficulty in the recovery phase.
- Depression is common.
- Support from ex-patients can be useful and, in the UK there is a national Guillain–Barré support group.

Critical illness polyneuropathy

This is a relatively newly recognized problem first described in 1984. It usually consists of severe axonal peripheral neuropathy arising in the context of people admitted to intensive care with severe sepsis and/or multiple trauma. In one study about half of individuals on intensive care for more than 7 days had documented evidence of peripheral neuropathy. The key points are:

- Recognize the syndrome.
- Ensure proper limb posture in order to minimize the risk of pressure sores and limb contractures.
- Use orthoses as necessary to maintain limbs in a neutral position.

- Rehabilitation usually follows the same lines as Guillain–Barré syndrome.
- Usually there is a good prognosis although recovery can take many weeks.
- A small proportion have long-term disability and thus will need long-term support.

Post-polio syndrome

Acute polio is now rare and has virtually been eradicated in the developed world and is significantly less common in developing countries. However, there are a still a large number of people who were affected by the disease, usually in their childhood. It is now increasingly recognized that late deterioration after polio can occur. The key points are:

- Post-polio syndrome usually occurs around 30–40 years after the acute illness.
- It is defined as the development of new neuromuscular symptoms (e.g. fatigue, muscle joint pain, weakness, increasing muscle wasting, etc.).
- It arises in the context of post-polio with no other determined cause.
- Sometimes the resulting disability can be disproportionate to the apparent minor change because of lack of functional reserve in people who are already disabled.
- Deterioration is usually slowly progressive. It is said that, on average, there is about 1% of loss of muscle strength each year. However, even a modest reduction in muscle strength of, say, 10% can be enough to produce severe further weakness in individuals already disabled after their acute polio.
- Fatigue can be a major symptom.
- Muscle pain, particularly cramping pain after exercise, can also be common.
- Aerobic training can improve muscle strength, at least to a limited degree.
- Treatment will focus on methods to assist weak limbs, such as the use of orthoses, mobility aids, wheelchairs, and environmental adaptation.

Hereditary motor and sensory neuropathies

There is an increasing genetic literature on a variety of hereditary motor and sensory neuropathies (HMSN). Slowly a number of genetic defects are being described, and it is quite likely in future years that some of these conditions will be treatable. However, at the moment there are no cures available for any form of HMSN. Rehabilitation will centre around:

- Proper diagnosis.
- Information and explanation regarding the nature of the condition.
- Description of the natural history so that appropriate future provisions can be made both by the treating rehabilitation team and the person and family.
- Possibility of genetic counselling for other members of the family.
- Physiotherapy advice regarding maintenance of a maximum degree of muscle strength.
- Appropriate prescription of orthoses and footwear to minimize the risks associated with soft tissue contracture.
- Regular chiropody is particularly important for those with sensory loss in the feet and hands.
- Provision of appropriate hand splints and other simple aids to daily living, such as adapted cutlery, pen holders, etc.
- Prescription of mobility aids, such as walking frames and wheelchairs and appropriate advice about driving and transport.
- Adaptation of the environment as necessary, such as ramps, lifts, hoists, assistive technology, etc.
- Surgical correction is sometimes necessary. This can involve Achilles tendon lengthening, plantar fasciotomy, posterior tibialis, long flexor and extensor tendon transfers, as well as the possibility of arthrodesis and osteotomies in order to preserve function and prevent complications.
- Progression is generally slow. Unnecessary complications should not be allowed to arise.

Finally, it should not be forgotten that some forms of peripheral neuropathy are quite treatable. This would include diabetic neuropathy where tight control of the diabetes is important. Rarer forms of neuropathies, such as vitamin B_{12} deficiency or vitamin E deficiency can improve dramatically with appropriate replacement therapy. The reader is referred to neurological texts for a definitive list of the causes of peripheral neuropathy and for a more detailed discussion of the various genetic forms of HMSN.

Brachial plexus injuries

Brachial plexus injuries are uncommon but nevertheless around 500 people in the UK suffer permanent disability each year, usually from traction injuries to the plexus. Brachial plexus injuries in childbirth still occur but they are becoming less common as obstetric practice improves. Road traffic accidents account for the great majority and indeed most are secondary to motorcycle accidents. The mean age is in the early 20s and the majority are males.

Individuals should be referred as soon as possible to a specialist centre where there is not only a good multidisciplinary rehabilitation team but also where expert surgical advice and treatment is obtainable.

Treatment will focus on:

- A very accurate diagnosis of the parts of the brachial plexus that have been damaged. This will involve a careful functional assessment often combined with neurophysiological investigation.
- If rupture or avulsion of the spinal nerves is suspected then surgical exploration should be carried out as soon as possible. There is a clear decline in long-term functional results if surgery is delayed. One series showed full return of function in individuals who were operated on within 3 weeks of the injury. However, the proportion of failures rose to over 60% in those operated on after 6 months. The nerves can be repaired either by grafting or nerve transfers.
- Specialist splints can be very useful and effectively restore function in individuals who do not make a full recovery after surgery. The following are particularly helpful:
  - An elbow lock splint is useful in the absence of active elbow control (C5 and C6 lesions).
  - A gauntlet splint is useful when there is major loss of function in the forearm and hand (C7, C8, and T1 lesions).
  - The flail arm splint is used when there is irreparable damage to the whole plexus (C5–T1 lesions). The flail arm splint will include an elbow hinge and a wrist platform to which can be attached various devices, such as split hook which is open and closed by a cable and operated from the opposite shoulder. Various other appliances can be attached to the flail arm device, such as attachments to aid activities of daily living around the house or in the garden. Some individuals can return to work using various splints attachments, such as pliers, sewing devices etc.

In summary the outlook is good for people with brachial plexus lesions as long as urgent referral is made to a specialist centre and the lesion is surgically explored and repaired as soon as possible. There is often much that can be done for those with residual arm and shoulder weakness. However, often the main disabling feature in the longer term is the presence of central neuropathic pain. This can be difficult to control. Treatment will focus on the use of anti-convulsants and/or tricyclic anti-depressants.

Epilepsy

Background

Epilepsy is common. Around 1% of the entire population will suffer at least one non-febrile seizure during their lives. The overall prevalence is around 5000 per 100 000 population with an incidence of around 50 per 100 000 population per annum. It is the most common disabling neurological condition in both adults and children. It is not a condition that is often seen by a multidisciplinary rehabilitation team. Epilepsy is intermittent and normally people function perfectly well in between fits without any associated disability. The management of epilepsy is normally restricted to a neurological service supported by specialist regional centres. Around the UK there are three residential establishments for people with persistent and intractable epilepsy.

Medical management

This section will specifically not deal with the classification of epilepsy or with the details of pharmacological anti-convulsant management. These are outside the remit of this book. However, some points can be made:

- Accurate diagnosis is essential. Diagnosis and investigation needs to rule out causes of secondary epilepsy which may lead to other potential treatments. Causes would include brain tumour, cerebrovascular disease, and a whole variety of inherited metabolic problems. Accurate diagnosis may obviously help prediction with natural history and prognosis and guide potential treatment.

- Accurate description of the type of epilepsy is important in order that appropriate anti-convulsant medication can be initiated if required.

- The great majority of individuals (over 80%) can be quite well controlled on a single anticonvulsant. Only a small minority will need combination anti-convulsant medication and such individuals need to be seen and monitored in a specialist centre.

- The most commonly prescribed anti-convulsants remain the well-established drugs, particularly carbamazepine, sodium valproate and phenytoin. Generally the newer drugs, such as gabapentin, vigabatrin, topiramate, lamotrigine, etc., are generally used as second-line treatment although some are now beginning to find a place as first-line options. On a global scale phenobarbitone is still used because it is cheap and effective, albeit with a very unsatisfactory range of side-effects. Monitoring of serum levels of anti-convulsants can be helpful to determine compliance and to maximize treatment, although not all anti-convulsants can be meaningfully measured in this way. The saturation kinetics of phenytoin need to be borne in mind as increases above, roughly, 300 mg daily can lead to dramatic increases in serum levels and consequent toxicity.

- It is important that individuals with epilepsy have long-term follow-up. Seizure type and frequency can change and there is a need for on-going monitoring of anti-convulsant efficacy and side-effects. Only around 6% of the UK epileptic population attend an epilepsy clinic. There is evidence that such people retain more information about their epilepsy

and are more satisfied with the service and support. A dedicated epilepsy service has a number of advantages, including:
- Expert management of the anti-convulsant regime.
- High-quality support from nursing staff who may be specifically trained in the management of epilepsy.
- Access to expert advice on such matters as driving, employment, etc.
- Psychological and counselling support.
- Support from local epilepsy groups.

Neuropsychological assessment and support

Most people with epilepsy have well-controlled seizures with no significant cognitive problems. However, some, particularly those with frequent or poorly controlled seizures, are at risk of cognitive and intellectual problems. This can be a result of the epilepsy itself, the underlying cause, or as a consequence of anti-convulsant medication.

The commonest difficulties are:
- Memory problems, particularly recent memory.
- Problems with information-processing speed.
- Problems with concentration or fatigue.
- Clinical anxiety and/or depression.

These neuropsychological problems need to be properly assessed and monitored and coping strategies put into place under the guidance of a clinical neuropsychologist. Psychologists can also be helpful in managing anxiety and depression, although sometimes medical input is required. Such symptoms can in themselves trigger seizures which in turn can lead to increased anxiety and thus more seizures, etc. Relaxation therapy can produce a significant reduction in seizure frequency in people prone to clinical anxiety.

Depression is probably best managed by cognitive strategies rather than anti-depressants as the latter can aggravate epilepsy.

Rarely, individuals with complex partial seizures can exhibit aggression during a seizure and the nature of the problem needs to be recognized and such seizures controlled as well as possible. Such individuals can often get into serious problems with the judicial system as a result of epileptic violence.

Social aspects of epilepsy

There are serious difficulties associated with the diagnosis of epilepsy, and there is often a profound effect on social, family, and work life.

Employment

Individuals with epilepsy are at a significantly higher risk of being unemployed compared with the general population. However, there is evidence that a trained epilepsy worker, such as a social worker or nurse, supporting the individual through job applications and interviews and visiting the employer can produce real benefit in terms of increased employment and retention rates. Advice needs to be given on occupations that are clearly inappropriate, such as flying, commercial diving, operating hazardous machinery, working at heights, and driving public service vehicles and commercial driving.

Driving

It is important for the epilepsy team to be fully acquainted with the complex area of driving legislation for people with epilepsy. This will vary from country to country. Driving is an essential part of modern society and an inability to drive can have a very significant impact on employment and social life. It can be vital for people living in rural situations. Inappropriate advice can lead to unnecessary disadvantage. At the present time in the UK people are allowed to drive as long as they have been seizure free for at least 1 year or attacks have only occurred whilst asleep for a period of at least 3 years. However, regulations change and the epilepsy team should be able to give full up-to-date advice from the Driving Vehicle Licensing Agency (DVLA) in Swansea. Responsibility for informing the DVLA falls with the licence holder and not the physician or the epilepsy team. However, the team do have an obligation to society as a whole to inform the DLVA if an individual is known to be driving and is thought to be a significant danger to society through, for example, frequent uncontrolled seizures.

Family

The family of the person with epilepsy needs to be involved in the whole process of diagnosis and on-going treatment. Support and guidance particularly need to be given to children. Such information could include:
- Full discussion about the nature of epilepsy.
- Knowledge of trigger factors, such as tiredness, alcohol, photosensitive triggers, etc.
- A good knowledge of appropriate first aid management during and immediately after a seizure.
- Full discussion on the broader social issues, such as social life, work, and driving.

Families with young children with epilepsy often have a difficult task in balancing normal risk-taking behaviour in children on the one hand and over-protection resulting in potential psychological problems and family strife on the other hand. Involvement of the whole family in appropriate counselling/support is essential.

Overall there is far more to epilepsy than management of anti-convulsant drugs. There is a clear need to involve an expert team in order to minimise disability and promote participation in society.

Dementia

General guidelines

Dementia usually falls within the province of the psychogeriatric team. However, dementia is not that uncommon in the younger population and is associated with a number of common neurologically disabling diseases, including:

- Parkinson's disease.
- Stroke.
- Multiple sclerosis.

There is also some tentative evidence that individuals with traumatic brain injury have a slightly higher risk of dementia in later life. Thus, the multidisciplinary rehabilitation team needs to be familiar with the approaches that can help the person with dementia.

Dementia is defined as a global impairment of function, including:

- Intellectual function.
- Memory.
- Higher perception.
- Language.
- Emotional and behavioural control.

An individual can function quite well in some domains whilst function very poorly in others. Thus, the first task is a full multidisciplinary assessment that will enable that particular person's strengths and weaknesses to be identified. Reassessment at frequent intervals is important as dementia is usually a progressive process and areas of initially preserved function can decline over time and different strategies may need to be adopted.

Most people with dementia are looked after in the community by friends and relatives and any rehabilitation process designed to support the person with dementia also needs to support their main carers. The carers must be involved in the assessment process, in designing appropriate strategies, and must be given long-term support. Many people with dementia can continue to live in the community and avoid the indignity and other problems associated with residential and nursing home care. However, others cannot be looked after by carers at home and will need residential admission. The staff in any residential environment obviously must be entirely familiar with the various strategies that can improve the lives of those with a dementing illness.

Rehabilitation in dementia is under-researched and many treatment approaches have not been properly evaluated. However, the next section outlines approaches that have shown to be helpful.

Helpful approaches

Environmental adaptation

People with dementia generally function better in a stable and familiar environment. This is often why people with dementia do quite well at home and, at least initially, do poorly if moved into a residential or nursing home. The physical environment is important and residential settings or rehabilitation units should do what they can to achieve a home-like atmosphere with a domestic style of furniture. People should have their own clothes and possessions in their immediate vicinity. Clear directions and signposting should be available. If individuals are less able to read then colour coding is often useful. For example, blue doors could mean bathrooms and red doors toilets. Basically as much effort as possible should be put into making the immediate environment familiar, routine, and non-threatening.

Stimulation activity

It seems clear that absence of sensory stimulation in some residential environments can compound behavioural disturbance. Some homes are characterized by drab colours, mass-produced furniture, and endless similar corridors. Attempts should be made to personalize the individual's own room as well as the home in general. However, in addition to this commonsense approach there is some, albeit limited, evidence that sensory stimulation including music, touch, taste, and smell can produce short-term benefit. Sensory stimulation can provide carers with some means of interaction. Some physical activity, within the confines of often frail people, and general occupation of time is useful. For example, it is important for the carers to be aware of the individual's previous lifestyle, hobbies, and interests and some attempt should be made to continue to interact with them by continuing with or discussing such interests.

Reminiscence

In dementia, at least in the early stages, individuals' past memories are usually reasonably intact. Thus, the use of a person's own past material, such as photo albums or newspaper cuttings and magazines, can act as prompts and triggers for memory. This can lead to an improved social interaction and probably reduces the risk of unnecessary depression, anxiety, and behavioural disturbance.

Reality orientation

Reality orientation (RO) aims to help the person with dementia continue to experience success and achievement as well as having an increased awareness of present reality. Regular RO sessions up to five times a week lasting about half an hour have shown to be beneficial in terms of orientation. Sessions will often be composed of a small group meeting on a regular basis and working on activities geared to increasing awareness of the immediate surroundings and of people around them. Informal RO will involve the staff and carers on a 24-h basis keeping the person in touch with current reality, such as the weather, day of the week, current news items, etc. Basically RO helps the person with dementia to continue to experience success and achievement and increase their awareness of present reality. There is evidence that many people with dementia are still able to learn and retain material under the right conditions. For example, a person can be successfully taught a number of face/name associations using prompting techniques that seek to avoid the occurrence of any errors. The absence of errors seems to improve learning.

Drug management

It is known that in people with Alzheimer's disease there is a deficit in cholinergic neurotransmission. The most useful approach seems to involve agents that inhibit the breakdown of acetylcholine by the enzyme acetyl cholinesterase resulting in an increase in the amount of acetylcholine available. Donepezil hydrochloride and rivastigmine are the first of the acetyl cholinesterase (ACE) inhibitors to be licensed for use in Alzheimer's disease. Some individuals on these drugs show improvements in cognition. Although the long-term impact of the drugs is yet to be established but it does seem clear that these drugs, and newer ones on the market, can apparently slow the progression of dementia, at least in some people.

In general terms psychotropic drugs should be avoided for the control of behaviour. However, occasionally marked symptoms of excitement, agitation, hallucination, or hostility can be responsive to neuroleptics. Side-effects can be a particular concern in the elderly population.

Sleep problems can be very troublesome, particularly for the family. Additional activity in the daytime can be useful by reducing the amount of daytime sleep and by establishment of a calming routine nearer bedtime. Sometimes a modest dose of a hypnotic, such as a benzodiazepine, may be necessary but once again should be avoided if at all possible. It should be remembered that older people do not actually need longer periods of sleep. If, in a nursing home, an individual is put to bed at 8.00 p.m. then it is not surprising that some individuals will then wake at 4.00 a.m. after 8 hours sleep!

Behavioural management

Behavioural management techniques have been described in Chapter 13. There is some evidence that appropriate behavioural management can produce some benefit for the demented person. Contingent reinforcement techniques in some residential environments have been shown to increase participation in daily activities and mobility as well as improvements in dressing and self-care tasks. Careful assessment of the individual based on the ABC principles (see Chapter 13) can sometimes lead to improvements in inappropriate behaviours and certainly seem worth trying as long as all the staff and/or the family are involved in the process.

Thus, there are a number of strategies which may well improve the lives of people with dementia and whilst not necessarily affecting the dementing process can certainly maximize quality of life both for the demented person and, as importantly, their family and carers.

Arthritis

Introduction

Arthritis is the largest cause of locomotor disability in developed countries. While the management of patients with arthritis is usually the responsibility of rheumatologists and orthopaedic surgeons, a rehabilitationist may be involved for mobility problems requiring therapy, for a wheelchair, or for an orthosis, and those with severe disabilities may require the help of a multiprofessional team, especially if they develop complications. It is therefore important to have a detailed knowledge of these diseases and rheumatological/musculoskeletal rehabilitation is thus included in specialist training in rehabilitation medicine. The following arthropathies will be described—rheumatoid arthritis, seronegative arthritis, and osteoarthritis.

Rheumatoid arthritis (RA)

Epidemiology

RA is the commonest inflammatory arthropathy. It has an incidence of 30/100 000 and a prevalence of 1000/100 000.

Presentation

- Classical symmetrical polyarthritis affecting small joints.
- Onward progression to involve larger joints.
- Basic lesion—chronic synovitis.
- Pain, swelling, tenderness, and loss of function in joints due to inflammation.
- Systemic disease affecting multiple target organs (see Table 26.1).

Significant structural disability is less common due to improvements in disease modification over the last 20 years. While life and quality of life can be prolonged, active rehabilitation is required to maintain abilities and function and prevent complications.

Natural history

The distribution of RA is different from that of osteoarthritis (OA):

- Chronic synovitis → pannus → joint destruction. Pathognomic feature— erosions of articular cartilage and underlying bone.
- Untreated → joint destruction, instability, and loss of function.
- Florid synovitis → further destroys cartilage and bone → overall joint disruption.

Rheumatoid disease therefore has a major impact on mobility and dexterity, as well as on general health. Patients with a positive rheumatoid factor—a circulating IgM immunoglobulin—are termed as seropositive and tend to have more aggressive disease (although this is not always the case), but 15% of patients have a seronegative rheumatoid arthritis. The non-articular complications of the disease risk the patient's health most and treatment is aimed at limiting the effects of the disease. There is a tendency for the disease is to burn itself out after 10 to 20 years and the residual disability at the end of this time depends on the degree of joint destruction and musculoskeletal deformity due to secondary osteoarthritis and damage to other target organs.

Surgery

General principles

Surgery is most effective during inactive phases of the disease and possibly after the disease has burnt itself out. The vulnerability of the cervical spine must be respected prior to intubation and all patients going to the operating theatre should wear a cervical collar to highlight this.

Synovectomy

Synovectomy is less commonly used now, but the aim is to reduce synovial thickening in the joint and thus to reduce the pain and loss of function in the joint. However, it often gave rise to marked stiffness and has been superceded by more effective medical management.

Table 26.1 Extra-articular manifestations of rheumatoid disease

Affected organ	Manifestation
Eyes	Sjögren's syndrome, keratoconjunctivitis sicca, scleritis
Heart	Pericarditis, myocarditis, valve abnormalities, Raynaud's phenomenon
Respiratory	Alveolitis, pleural effusions, nodules, crico-arytenoid joint arthritis
Blood vessels	Vasculitis producing micro-infarcts, rashes, neuropathy, ulcers etc.
Skin	Rash, ulcers, nerves, vasculitic lesions
CNS	Compression syndromes, sensorimotor neuropathies, encephalomyelitis
Spinal cord	Transverse myelitis, cord compression
Gut	Dysphagia from Sjögren's syndrome, bowel infarcts (drug-induced gastrointestinal problems)
Kidneys	Glomerulonephritis, immune complex disease, amyloidosis
Blood	Anaemia of chronic inflammation, Felty's syndrome, thrombocytosis
Reticuloendothelial system	Lymphadenopathy, Felty's syndrome, non-specific hepatitis
General	Nodule formation, e.g. in subcutaneous tissues over areas of pressure

Arthrodesis and arthroplasty

This is a highly effective way to reduce joint pain, but has now been superceded by joint replacement, particularly in the hips and knees, as its legacy is significant resultant disability. Hip, knee, and shoulder arthroplasties have become very effective and the first two are now commonly carried out. Elbow replacement is becoming increasingly possible, but is still at a relatively early stage in its development. The ankle joint is a difficult joint to replace and arthrodesis here is more useful at the present time. Most people can cope quite well with a stiff ankle.

Other procedures

Carpal tunnel decompression is carried out in many rheumatoid patients. Surgery to the spine, and in particular to the lower part of the neck, may have to be considered where cervical myelopathy is a danger, and fusion of the cervical spine may be required at both the atlanto-occipital and atlanto-axial levels and in the lower cervical spine.

Important issues in the rehabilitation of patients with RA

What do we need to know about rheumatoid patients prior to setting up a rehabilitation programme? The following specific issues have an impact on the life of the patient and on his or her rehabilitation:

• Fatigue.
• Distribution of joint pain and stiffness.
• Skeletal deformities.

Rheumatoid arthritis (RA) (*continued*)

- Soft tissue swelling.
- Mobility and daily activity.
- Functional performance and capacity for improvement in performance.
- Psychosocial problems.
- Environmental issues.

Diurnal variations in performance are important, and early morning stiffness is not only a marker of disease activity but has an impact on the patient's lifestyle. Underpinning the rehabilitation process is the need for effective medication, e.g. non-steroidal anti-inflammatory drugs (NSAIDs) and disease-modifying agents.

Control of pain and physical treatment
- Acute joint flares are severe and debilitating but show rapid resolution with treatment.
- Chronic pain affects the joints, muscles, and limbs and leads to significant disability, including depression and exhaustion.
- Physical treatment: Cold packs and hot packs, heat for stiff joints, electricity, laser treatment, transcutaneous electrical nerve stimulation (TENS) and acupuncture are used along with exercise, both on dry land and in water. Cold packs should be applied for about 10 min to swollen, stiff, and painful joints and pain reduction occurs through reduction of muscle spasm. Hydrotherapy delivers heat and exercises joints. Ultrasound penetrates skin to a depth of about 5 cm and has analgesic properties and can increase the distensibility of tissue. Several studies have reported the efficacy of acupuncture for the relief of joint pain in RA, more comprehensive studies of the effectiveness of physical treatments are required.

Orthoses
Orthoses are used to settle rest joints during a flare and have been described in greater detail in Chapter 12.
- Hand splints: there are four main functions to be addressed when considering an orthosis for the hand:
  - Power grip: when the wrist is slightly extended and when the fingers are flexed at the metacarpo-phalangeal and interphalangeal joints.
  - Pinchgrip: when the thumb and index finger are in contact.
  - Key grip: when there is opposition of the thumb to the side of the index finger.
  - Hook grip: e.g. allows a suitcase or handbag to be carried on flexed metacarpophalangeal and interphalangeal joints—the wrist is in a neutral position and the thumb is not involved.
- Lower limb splints: primarily immobilize and support joints; these are addressed in Chapter 12.
- Collars: the wearing of collars and spinal supports always raises controversy. C1/2 instability must be addressed and prevented, so good posture is necessary, particularly while the patient is asleep. Surgical stabilization of the spine should be considered if there is more than 8 mm of subluxation between the odontoid peg and the

atlas, and the wearing of a Halo splint should be considered at about 6 mm. A rigid neck brace with chin support (e.g. a SOMI type brace) is recommended for physical activity in which flexion and extension may occur. Other collars, such as the Philadelphia collar, are also available; this is better tolerated because it in fact allows more flexion and extension.

Drug treatment

This falls outside the remit of this text. Following gold and penicillamine, sulphasalazine and methotrexate have had wide usage. Hydroxychloroquine is indicated in patients with a positive antinuclear antigen and rheumatoid factor who express the HLA-D3 gene. Intra-articular and systemic steroids are also of use in preventing either local or generalized joint flares respectively. They should be accompanied by a period of rest followed by mobilization of the affected part. Biologic treatment, such as anti-tumour necrosis factor (infliximab) and monoclonal antibody are now potent treatments, which are revolutionizing rheumatological practice and outcomes for patients.

Joint protection and education

The most important factor in education of the patient relates to their lifestyle. Table 26.2 considers some of the decision that are required in ensuring that quality of life can be maintained.

Outcome measures

- Disease activity: control correlates with low C-reactive protein and erythrocyte sedimentation rate (ESR).
- Joint pain and tenderness: Ritchie Articular Index.
- Number of erosions on x-rays: Larsen score.
- Global score: this is elusive, as in many other conditions; overall assessment is a combination of pathological markers, impairment scores, and activity and participation measures.

Table 26.2 Lifestyle decisions with RA

Is sufficient time given for personal activities of daily living?

Are disability aids required for your own personal care or domestic activities?

Is help required for personal care or domestic activities?

What is your role within the family and among significant others? (has this changed due to the arthritis?)

What help is required for you to maintain your employment/occupational activity?

What aspects of activities can you ignore or delegate to others?

What must be done today, this week, this month, this year?

Is time for leisure, recreation, and rest incorporated into your daily/weekly plan?

What arrangements are being made for significant events, e.g. partnership/marriage, having a family, retirement etc.

Seronegative arthritis

Seronegative arthritis is a term used to describe a family of inflammatory arthritides in which there is a genetic linkage to the HLA-B27 antigen between the conditions and between family members. It is not unknown for different types of seronegative arthritis to occur in members of the same family.

The different seronegative arthritides are discussed below, but they all have the following general features:

- They affect the large weight-bearing joints, sacroiliac joints, and spine.
- They have a relationship to diseases of the gastrointestinal tract, the genitourinary system, the eyes, and the skin.

Characteristics

- Associated with a 'boggy' synovitis of large weight-bearing joints (ankles and knees).
- Does not usually give rise to major joint deformities (contrast RA).
- Associated with back pain, improves with activity, but returns with inactivity.
- Stiffness in the morning and following inactivity.
- Include conjunctivitis, urethritis, colitis, skin conditions (e.g. psoriasis and keratoderma blenorrhagica).
- Pain responds to NSAIDs; corticosteroids tend to be unhelpful.
- The condition usually burns out, but is variable in its length.
- A constant feature is negativity of the rheumatoid factor.

Ankylosing spondylitis (AS)

An arthritis affecting young men aged 15 to 30, which is active for 10–20 years. It invariably starts off as a sacroiliitis with low back pain and may proceed to involve the lumbar spine, the thoraco-lumbar junction, and the cervical spine. Stiffness is the key symptom, along with pain, and the spine may become so stiff that ventilation is reduced. Peripheral joints can also be involved and there can be stiffness of other musculoskeletal structures. In spinal disease, the maintenance of a good truncal position and of hip movements is vital for continued personal functioning and repeated measures of chest expansion and lumbar flexion using Schöber's test and a wall to tragus distance are required:

- *Schöber's test*: The patient should be standing. A mark is made on the back at the level of the iliac crest (L4 vertebral body). Another mark is made 5 cm above this, and a third is made 10 cm below. The patient is then asked to touch his toes and the distance between the second and third marks are measured. In a normal person there is a ≥7 cm difference between standing and bending forward.
- *Wall to tragus test*: The patient stands against a wall and the distance is simply measured from the wall to the tragus of the ear.

Sacroiliac joint tenderness is measured by direct palpation, and it is also important to measure and document extension and flexion of the hip joints. Preservation of hip extension is the key to maintaining functional mobility in AS. Cervical spine movement should also be preserved to avoid late neurological compression.

A typical stiff spine may ensue without a programme of regular exercise. It is important that exercise is maintained throughout the course of the disease and smokers must be actively discouraged from continuing their habit. The combination of restricted ventilation and the loss of parenchymal elasticity and ciliary movement caused by smoking comprise a potentially lethal combination.

Psoriatic arthritis (PsA)

Psoriatic arthritis is a seronegative arthritis associated with the skin condition psoriasis. It is usually associated with pitting of the nails, which is an indicator that the arthritis is related to the psoriasis. As psoriasis itself is so common, it can occur in combination with seropositive rheumatoid arthritis and it is important to differentiate between RA and psoriatic arthritis. It presents in three forms:

- A mild peripheral polyarthritis, usually affecting the distal interphalangeal joints.
- A severe polyarthritis, causing arthritis mutilans—rapidly progressive, grossly destructive disease. Associated with florid skin disease. The small joints of the hands are involved and destroyed.
- A spinal arthritis, closely identified with AS. Sacroiliitis occurs, but is not necessarily symmetrical.

Table 26.3 Treatment plan for some seronegative arthritides

Disease	Stage	Treatment
AS	Early and mild disease	Assessment on review in all cases. NSAIDs. Physiotherapy (exercises and general fitness training, incl. swimming). Advice about smoking, lifestyle, work, etc.
	Moderate disease ± peripheral arthritis	NSAIDs.? Disease modifiers (sulphasalazine, methotrexate, anti-TNF)? Injection of selected peripheral joints. Exercises as above. General measures to address disability and handicap
	Late disease	Above plus addressing functioning and participation (F&P) issues
PsA	Mild peripheral disease	As for early/mild AS plus treatment of psoriasis
	Progressive peripheral disease	As for early/mild AS plus injection of selected joints, disease-modifying drugs. Surgery to appropriate joints. Address F&P issues
RD		NSAIDs. Antibiotic cover for acute attacks. Sulphasalazine for persistent disease. Inject appropriate joints and/or enthesopathy. Education on multiple sexual partners and on bowel infection. Therapy and orthoses as required. Surgery if necessary

Seronegative arthritis (*continued*)

Reiter's disease (RD)

Reiter's disease classically affects sexually active young men and women. It starts with a urethritis or with bowel inflammation, followed several days later by a conjunctivitis and 5 to 7 days thereafter by an acute arthritis (either a unilateral sacroiliitis or, more often, affecting one or two large weight-bearing joints, e.g. ankle and knee). An enthesopathy (e.g. plantar fasciitis), skin lesions (e.g. keratoderma blenorrhagica), mucosal lesions in the mouth and on the genitals, and a circinate balanitis in males may also occur. The urethritis is often non-specific, but can occur after gonococcal urethritis and *Yersinia*, *Campylobacter*, *Shigella*, and *Salmonella* have all been implicated.

Post-colitic arthritis

Both ulcerative colitis and Crohn's disease are associated with arthritis, which takes on a similar picture to both the peripheral and spinal disease seen in psoriatic arthritis. Flares come and go with attacks of bowel disease. Control of the underlying bowel disease usually leads to control of the joint disease.

Reactive arthritis or sexually acquired reactive arthritis (SARA)

Similar to the above conditions in presentation, but is associated with a non-specific urethritis or a non-specific colitis and is a term often used for incomplete features of the above conditions. The response to treatment is similar and the arthritic condition is usually self-limiting.

Treatment

Table 26.3 illustrates some treatment plans for seronegative arthritides.

Osteoarthritis (OA)

Osteoarthritis is a common degenerative joint disease with an unknown incidence which is estimated at about 200 per 100 000 population per year for hip and knee osteoarthritis. The prevalence is 3.8% at the knee and 1.3% at the hip, and osteoarthritis is the most common joint disease in the world. Its impact is therefore huge. It is not actually one disease but represents the endpoint of a series of insults to the joint. The impression of osteoarthritis is that it is due to wear and tear, but it is not a condition of relentless progression. It is not in itself a systemic disease and its effects are purely local—an imbalance appears between a joint's ability to withstand stresses and the actual forces on the joint. Genetic and biochemical factors obviously play a part in loss of articular cartilage. There is a failure of the articular cartilage matrix which damages its surface and activates chondrocytes. Repair defects occur resulting in proteoglycan loss, collagen damage, and finally cartilage thinning and loss. Cartilage nutrition is also impaired through a failure of synovial fluid. Primary and secondary forms exist, and the latter can occur as a result of longstanding stresses on a joint. Altered biomechanics from anatomical defects can give rise to forces on a joint over a concentrated area rather than over the whole of the joint surface and the joint will inevitably wear at this point.

Primary osteoarthritis

Primary osteoarthritis is common and occurs in middle-aged and elderly people. It is a mild inflammatory condition:

- Characterized by its distribution through joints and the presence of Heberden's nodes on distal interphalangeal joints (DIPJs).
- Bouchard's nodes also exist but no features of rheumatoid disease.
- Primary OA classically affects the knees, hips, DIPJs, first carpometacarpal joint, lower cervical spine and first metatarsophalangeal joint.
- Leads to pain and swelling in joints and to the need for eventual hip and knee joint replacement in more severe cases.
- Small rise in the ESR and C-reactive protein. Negative rheumatoid factor.

Secondary osteoarthritis

There are several types of secondary osteoarthritis:

- *Developmental*: hypermobility syndromes due to anatomical defects or biochemical faults; congenital dislocation of the hip; Perthes' disease; epiphyseal dysplasias.
- *Infective/septic*: local inflammation or more commonly from a distant septic focus.
- *Inflammatory*: following haemarthrosis etc.
- *Metabolic*: ochronosis, haemochromatosis, acromegaly, crystal arthritis, etc.
- *Mechanical*: obesity, direct trauma, previous joint surgery, longstanding deformity.

Clinical features

Clinical features are listed in Table 26.4.

Management

Pain and stiffness should be controlled by analgesia, and acute flares of joint disease may be managed by rest, physiotherapy, and/or local injections of corticosteroids or hyalouronic acid. In chronic pain, anti-depressant drugs may be required to modify the patient's response and supplement analgesics. The Bone and Joint Decade and The European League Against Rheumatism (EULAR) have defined some indications of the impact of medications in osteoarthritis, which include measurement of pain on a visual analogue scale, patient's global assessment, and walking time. Walking and other mobility aids are important, and disability equipment can certainly help osteoarthritic people at home. Surgery has transformed the outcome for hip, knee, and shoulder OA and ankle prostheses are being developed.

Complications

- Limb deformity resulting in loss of function (e.g. mobility) and tendon injury.
- Falls and fractures from joint instability.
- Nerve compression (e.g. spinal cord and root compression in canal stenosis, carpal tunnel syndrome).
- Vascular compression (e.g. avascular necrosis of bone, deep vein thrombosis from Baker's cyst).
- Mood changes from chronic pain.
- Complications of surgery.

Table 26.4 Clinical features of OA

Symptoms	Signs
Post-activity stiffness	Joint tenderness
Mild early morning stiffness	Muscle weakness
Pain on activity and at night	Periarticular soft tissue swelling, bony enlargement
Loss of joint function	Joint effusion
Joint swelling	Joint crepitus
Instability	Loss of joint range of movement, instability
Decreased walking speeds	Gait abnormalities
Normal general health	Imaging abnormalities, normal laboratory investigations

Spinal pain and soft tissue rheumatism

Low back and neck pain are common and may result from abnormalities occurring within the vertebrae, the intervertebral discs, the facet joints, or the ligaments, or from the spinal canal and the nerve roots themselves. Pain may be referred from distant sites, such as the abdomen, and in some cases may be functional or psychogenic in nature.

Acute back pain

Causes of acute back pain may be:
- Muscular or ligamentous strain.
- Intervertebral disc prolapse.
- Facet joint dysfunction.
- Bony trauma.
- Acute inflammatory disease or infection (joint or bony).
- Tumours.

Acute pain *de novo* does not usually present to a physician in rehabilitation medicine and this topic is better addressed in rheumatological and orthopaedic texts. The treatment of back pain has been described in the Clinical Standards Advisory Group (CSAG) guidelines and bed rest is nowadays not recommended for acute simple low back pain. Short-term rest may be useful for some patients in the case of intervertebral disc prolapse, when pain may be referred to the leg by nerve root entrapment. When this occurs in a true spinal root distribution it is known as sciatica, but the term should not be applied to other referred pain in the leg and back.

It is important to identify the patient's description of pain. He or she may often refer to buttock pain as hip pain and, unless pinned down, will be quite vague about the distribution of any leg pain. Knowledge of the spine's anatomy and of the typical radiation patterns of pain is therefore important.

Management

Acute back pain usually resolves spontaneously after a few days or weeks. Investigation is required to rule out underlying inflammation or neoplasia:
- Analgesics.
- Imaging in simple acute back pain is usually unhelpful, but may give an indication of previous underlying disease such as lumbar spondylosis or osteoporosis.
- Prolonged bed rest not advised.
- Leg pain and sciatica may be helped by a lumbar or caudal epidural injection.
- Acute exacerbation of facet joint pain, in which there is a local tenderness of one and no more than two joints, may be eased by local infiltration of corticosteroid and local anaesthetic.
- Exercises such as Maitland's and McKenzie mobilizations have been shown to be useful, but no more effective than other forms of physical treatment. The aim is to relieve the pressure on the spinal structures and rest and cessation of the incriminating factors will usually settle the situation.
- Use of isokinetic devices to help restore mechanical function appears to be useful, but needs further study.

Chronic back pain

Causes

Causes of chronic back pain include:

- Posture.
- Facet joint pain.
- Short leg syndrome.
- Lumbar spondylosis.
- Degenerative disc disease.
- Spondylolisthesis and spondylolysis.
- Diffuse idiopathic skeletal hyperostosis.
- Spinal stenosis.

Posture

Prolonged poor posture alters the normal curve of the spine and stresses the structures therein.

Short leg syndrome

Unequal leg lengths tilt the pelvis, producing a scoliosis in the spine and straining ligaments and joints. Correcting the difference in leg length may be helpful.

Prolapsed intervertebral disc

The particular disc which is prolapsed will affect the symptoms (Table 27.1).

Facet joint pain

This is a well-defined back pain syndrome associated with lumbar spondylosis. Pain is experienced on extension of the spine, both in an upright position and in sitting, and can be provoked on bending forwards. The pain often radiates to the buttock or into the sacrum and may extend down the leg but rarely extends beyond the knee. This is not nerve root pain.

Spondylosis

Dysfunction of vertebral structures causes a chronic low-grade pain. This is the end result of degenerative changes in the spine and occurs at points of movement of the spine (facet joints and vertebral bodies).

Spondylolisthesis and spondylolysis

This is a displacement of one vertebra on another—usually an anterior movement of a vertebra above on the one below, but posterior movement of the vertebra above on that below can also occur and is referred to as retrolisthesis. Spondylolysis occurs when the spondylolisthesis is caused by a defect in the pars interarticularis in the vertebral lamina. The symptoms are very similar to that of facet joint pain.

Spinal stenosis

Chronic disease of the spine can cause narrowing of the spinal canal or foramen following recurrent disc prolapse and loss of disc height, or as a result of facet joint arthritis impinging into the spinal canal. Back and leg pain occur with physical activity and then settle at rest in most patients. It is also found that flexion of the spine relieves the symptoms and walking up hills and going up stairs is often more comfortable than on the flat or going downhill. MRI is diagnostic at confirming the level of narrowing and a laminectomy is the treatment of choice.

Table 27.1 Prolapsed intervertebral disc

Disc prolapse	Affected nerve root	Loss of reflex	Dermatome	Typical muscle weakness
L3/4	L4	Knee jerk	Anterior aspect of knee and medial aspect of the lower leg down to the ankle	Quadriceps, part of tibialis anterior, tibialis posterior
L4/5	L5		Postero-lateral aspect of thigh, lateral aspect of lower leg, dorsum and medial aspect of foot including the medial 3 1/2 toes	Foot dorsiflexors and evertors. Tibialis posterior
L5/S1	S1	Ankle jerk	Small strip of posterior aspect of thigh and posterior aspect of calf, heel and lateral aspect of foot including lateral 1 1/2 toes	Foot plantar flexors, lateral hamstrings and thigh abductors (gluteus maximus)

Chronic back pain (*continued*)

Specific management
Table 27.2 gives details of management of chronic back pain depending on the cause.

Pain management
Patient education and the development of a realistic approach to lifestyle management are important. Treat acute painful exacerbations. A suitable regimen of analgesics and therapies is required for background pain. Direct management should be related to to social and occupational needs rather than a search for a cure.

Management of chronic pain is discussed in Chapter 11.

The patient should be taught mild, gentle, but effective exercise by a physiotherapist to improve muscle strength and to mobilize the spine. Thereafter, the patient should be expected to continue the exercises, particularly during quiescent periods. Warm water exercises in a local swimming pool are valuable in providing heat and a medium in which exercise can be done.

Lifestyle management is the rewarding aspect of rehabilitation. Psychological advice may identify the key issues producing the symptoms in some patients with clear instructions on how to manage daily routines and deal with acute exacerbations. Patients and relatives must be given consistent messages for successful outcomes. Therapy should be reserved for acute exacerbations, for which there should be clear indications. The specialist team should also involve the primary care team, social services and the disability employment adviser. Alterations to the home, workplace and transportation are important, and back pain sufferers should be encouraged to take up activities which will not cause particular difficulties for their symptoms.

Table 27.2 Management of chronic back pain

Cause of pain	Management
Posture	Analgesics; treat the underlying cause
Short leg syndrome	Correct the leg length difference with either an insole or shoe raise
Prolapsed disc	Most settle spontaneously with rest, but the biomechanical effect on the facet joints must be addressed. Discectomy for intractable nerve root compression
Facet joint pain	Analgesia; joint injection
Spondylosis	Analgesia for acute pain, hydrotherapy for stiffness (see Chapter 11)
Spondylolisthesis/lysis	Treatment usually conservative. Immobilization of the spine for bad symptoms or for nerve root compression. Spinal fusion may be a definitive procedure
Spinal stenosis	Laminectomy is the treatment of choice

Neck pain

Neck pain is common and the principles of management are similar to those for managing back pain. Acute exacerbations are a common feature of chronic neck pain. Symptom duration following injury depends on severity, but should settle within a few weeks in the absence of disruption of the ligamentous structures to the spine. Neck pain of mechanical origin usually produces asymmetric restriction of movement, whereas neck pain of inflammatory origin (e.g. rheumatoid disease, ankylosing spondylitis) tends to be symmetrical.

Clinical features

- Acute exacerbations: most last for no more than a few days and are often associated with some unaccustomed activity, awkward posture, or injury.
- Pain and stiffness: back of lower neck, radiates to occiput, down spine, shoulders/down arms. Usually aggravated by movement of the neck and relieved by rest.
- Nerve root compression may occur, most commonly in the C7 dermatome.
- Whiplash injury: in whiplash injury anterior neck pain may be present for several months. The absence of nerve root involvement and a full range of neck movements on active and passive examination would suggest complete resolution of the neck pain symptoms. These would not be expected to persist for more than 2 years or give rise to subsequent degenerative change.

Symptoms in *mechanical causes* are intermittent with pain confined to an articular and dural distribution. Neurological features confined to a single root. *Worrying signs* are constant or progressive symptoms and bilateral neurological signs or those involving more than one nerve root.

Tables 27.3 and 27.4 give more details of symptoms, signs and the relationship of pain distribution to the site of the problem.

Treatment

Analgesics and rest, perhaps with use of a soft collar to maintain a neutral position, can be helpful. There is considerable debate about whether collars are helpful or harmful. There is no doubt that they have a place in providing some short-term relief for patients with acute exacerbations of chronic neck pain and their main benefit comes from intermittent use, even in some cases nocturnal usage. Collars also have their place for short-term use after acute injuries, but in the long term they can produce stiffness and loss of movement in the spine, which can allow the patient to develop unnecessary longer-lasting symptoms. If there is a risk of neurological injury, then a collar is mandatory to restrict movements. They are also of importance in patients with severe erosive rheumatoid disease going for surgery, even if they do not have gross cervical spine disease. This alerts the anaesthetist to the risk of cord damage from neck extension

Table 27.3 Neck pain: symptoms and signs

Problem	Symptoms	Signs
Articular	Intermittent neck pain	Asymmetrical restriction of neck movement
Dural	Occiput, vertex, scapula, shoulder and interscapular pain	Pain may occur on shoulder adduction or external rotation, but pain on forced lateral flexion of cervical spine
Nerve root	Severe pain in appropriate dermatome	Weakness and sensory impairment in affected nerve root distribution, abnormal reflex if necessary

during intubation. The aim is to restrict neck movements to about one-third, and while rigid collars can achieve reduction to about 10% they are cumbersome and uncomfortable to wear. They should thus be reserved for patients at risk of neurological compression.

Physical treatment

Physiotherapy and chiropracty are commonly performed. Traction can be used when root pain occurs in either a lying or sitting position. There is evidence to support the use of manual techniques over exercise in decreasing pain and maintaining range of movement. Mobilization exercises and manipulation are also performed where cervical joints are repeatedly pressed through their ranges of movement. Manipulation is simply a more energetic and aggressive form of mobilization, but older patients should not generally be subjected to it (Braddom, R.L. *Physical Medicine and Rehabilitation* 2nd edn. 2001. W.B. Saunders, Philadelphia). Patients with chronic pain may also respond to both TENS and acupuncture, which have a useful carry-over effect after use.

Medication

Analgesics and anti-inflammatories are the mainstay of treatment in acute neck pain (see Chapter 11 for more detail). There is no good evidence for the effectiveness of the latter in mechanical and degenerative disease, but the reality is that patients feel that they are helpful. For the most part, patients are usually managed with a combination of analgesics and physical treatments, but in some cases this is not enough. Mood changes quite quickly on the realization that the pain has started to persist and the addition of a tricyclic anti-depressant is helpful. The evidence points to the latter being more effective than other types, although in reality both these and selective serotonin uptake inhibitors have wide usage. Gabapentin is being increasingly used for a wide variety of pain and there is good evidence for its effect on neurogenic pain. Topical medication is not helpful in neck pain, as creams do not have enough penetration to even reach down to the underlying muscles.

Neck pain (*continued*)

Surgery

In degenerative disease, surgery is only indicated for cord or nerve root compression, or for instability of the spine where a fusion is required. This may be done through a posterior or anterior approach, but the latter is favoured for degenerative or disc disease at the present time with the Cloward procedure being the operation of choice.

Because neck pain can become chronic and very disabling, many other associated features can develop, which are discussed further in Chapter 11.

Table 27.4 Neck pain: pain distribution

Root	Pain distribution	Muscle weakness	Tendon reflex
C2	Occiput radiating over head to forehead neck, jaw, and cheek		
C3			
C4	Trapezius and upper medial border of the scapula		
C5	Shoulder tip, lateral side of the upper arm	Supraspinatus, infraspinatus, deltoid, biceps	Biceps
C6	Front of arm, lateral aspect of elbow and radial border of forearm down to thumb	Biceps, supinator	Supinator
C7	Middle of anterior and posterior aspects of forearm, middle, and ring fingers	Triceps, wrist flexors	Triceps
C8	Ulnar aspect of forearm and hand, ring and little finger	Wrist and finger flexors, thumb flexors	
T1	Medial aspect of elbow. Upper pectoral and mid-scapula areas	Intrinsic hand muscles	
T2	Medial aspect of upper arm and axilla		

Shoulder pain

The upper limb is suspended from the trunk by muscular attachments and thus any condition affecting muscular strength or function may cause pain affecting the *shoulder* (glenohumeral) *joint* itself, the *acromio-clavicular joint* or the *rotator cuff group of muscles*. In addition, degenerative disease in the neck, brachial plexus dysfunction, trapezius muscle spasm, and diaphragmatic and pericardial conditions may cause referred shoulder pain, but these will not be considered in detail. The skin around the shoulder is supplied by the C5 root, which will lead to shoulder muscle (rotator cuff) weakness when damaged, as well as sensory disturbance over the point of the shoulder.

Pain classically occurs on movement or when lying on the affected side at night. The 'painful arc syndrome' causes discomfort as the shoulder is raised in abduction and, as the movement continues, the pain then disappears. A shoulder must keep moving to maintain function and a fall may produce supraspinatus tendon damage and extreme pain, such that the patient stops moving the limb. The restriction of movement can lead very quickly on to a true frozen shoulder, i.e. an adhesive capsulitis. Three distinct syndromes exist in the painful shoulder, which are as follows.

Rotator cuff lesions

Rotator cuff lesions may occur in degenerative change or following an injury, e.g. falling onto an outstretched hand. A rotator cuff syndrome may occur as a result of vascular changes and mechanical factors affecting normal muscular and tendon function which produces pain. Over time, the space between the acromion process and the glenohumeral joint diminishes, leading particularly to restriction of the supraspinatus tendon and an impingement syndrome. The various elements of the rotator cuff syndrome are discussed below:

Supraspinatus tendinitis
Supraspinatus tendinitis affects the supraspinatus mechanism closest to its insertion into the greater tuberosity, and pain and limitation of active and passive abduction are characteristic. A painful arc occurs on abduction between 90° and 120°. The pain may be increased by resisting abduction of the arm in the first 15° of movement by placing the examiner's hand on the elbow and asking the patient to abduct the arm against the examiner's hand on the elbow. Some cases occur acutely and are associated with calcium deposits (seen on X-ray). Injection into the subacromial bursa is the medical treatment of choice.

Infraspinatus/subscapularis tendinitis
Although less common than supraspinatus tendinitis, these two lesions give distinctive features. Both cause pain on abduction of the arm, but the former gives rise to pain on external rotation of the arm and the latter to pain on internal rotation of the arm. The former is more common in sportsmen than other lesions of the rotator cuff. Table 27.5 details the rotator cuff muscles.

Table 27.5 Rotator cuff muscles

Muscle	Action	Innervation
Deltoid	Abduction and flexion of arm 15–90°	Axillary nerve
Supraspinatus	Abduction of arm 0–15° and 90° upwards	Suprascapular nerve
Infraspinatus	External rotation of arm	Suprascapular nerve
Subscapularis	Internal rotation of arm	Suprascapular nerve
Serratus anterior	Protraction of arm	Long thoracic nerve
Biceps brachii long head	Forearm supination, elbow/shoulder flexion	Musculocutaneous nerve
Pectoralis major	Adduction of arm	Long thoracic nerve
Teres major and minor	Adduction of arm	Axillary nerve
Latissimus dorsi	Adduction of arm from 60°	
Rhomboids	Shoulder extension	

Bicipital tendinitis
This produces pain anteriorly on the shoulder in the area where the bicipital tendon passes through the groove in the humeral head to attach in the coracoid process. Local injection is helpful.

Subacromial bursitis
This somewhat non-specific term describes a rotator cuff problem where the specific tendon lesion is not readily identifiable. The pain is evident on shoulder abduction and flexion and both may be restricted. Stressing the individual tendons may not produce intense pain in one area more than in others. The most common feature is a painful arc around 60–120° of abduction.

Adhesive capsulitis—frozen shoulder

Frozen shoulder occurs following trauma, following rotator cuff lesions, or following immobility from other causes, e.g. stroke, chest surgery, and pathology (myocardial infarction, pericarditis, and particularly sternal splits). It may be spontaneous and is more common in diabetics. The essential feature is an inflamed glenohumeral capsule, which eventually shrinks and thickens, thus restricting movement. Abduction is restricted in common with rotator cuff lesions, but the pathognomonic feature is loss of external rotation. Early treatment is important, as a secondary reflex sympathetic dystrophy can occur leading to a useless arm and hand, which will be very difficult to treat.

Acromioclavicular joint lesions

Acromioclavicular joint lesions develop in people in their 40s and 50s due to joint degeneration. There is joint tenderness and pain on stressing flexion and abduction of the arm between 60 and 90°. Radiographs show loss of joint space and possibly osteophytes, which may cause an impingement syndrome by inferior projection.

Shoulder pain (*continued*)

Treatment of shoulder pain

Treatment of these lesions is essentially with analgesics and physiotherapy to mobilize the joint. NSAIDs are of little use and it may be necessary to use quite strong analgesics to allow sleep. Rotator cuff lesions may respond to an injection of steroid and local anaesthetic into the sub-acromial bursa and adhesive capsulitis responds by similar infiltration into the glenohumeral joint itself. If rotator cuff lesions persist and are clearly due to impingement, it may be necessary after MR or ultra sound scanning to decompress the space surgically. Injection of the acromioclavicular joint can be very effective if the pain emanates from there. Similarly, the distal end of the clavicle may require removal in persistent severe acromioclavicular joint pain. The principle of treating adhesive capsulitis is to mobilize the joint physically and to utilize injections to allow physical treatment to be taken further. If this is not possible, manipulation of the joint under anaesthetic has no proven effect, but is useful in some patients as long as an intensive series of physiotherapy treatments is planned for 5 days immediately after the procedure. The prognosis is in fact very good for all these lesions.

Lateral humeral epicondylitis (tennis elbow) and medial humeral epicondylitis (golfer's elbow)

These are two annoying conditions in people over the age of 40—thought to be part of an upper limb overuse syndrome resulting from excessive tension on the common forearm extensor and flexor muscles respectively, which results in localized tenderness and pain on gripping and twisting the hand. They often prevent function of the hand, particularly in lifting weights and may be associated with neck pain:

* Tennis elbow:
  – Tender lateral humeral epicondyle.
  – Epicondylar pain on resisting wrist or finger extension supporting the arm (straight elbow).
  – Forced pronation of the forearm with the elbow straight also produces pain.
* Golfer's elbow:
  – Tender medial humeral epicondyle.
  – Epicondylar pain on resisting wrist or finger flexion supporting the arm (straight elbow).
  – Pain on resisted supination less reliable.
  – Sensory symptoms do not typically occur.

Atypical feature of epicondylitis include:
* Bilateral symptoms and signs, or the presence of both golfer's and tennis elbow.
* No epicondylar tenderness.
* Paraesthesiae in the arm and painful limitation of neck movements, associated with nerve root disturbance.
* Failure to respond to local injection or occurrence within a week or two of injection.
* Clinical or radiological evidence of arthritis at the elbow.

Treatment

Physical treatment is usually helpful in mild cases. No one particular treatment has been shown to be superior to another. An epicondylitis clasp worn reasonably tightly around the upper forearm just below the common extensor or common flexor origin can protect the common muscular origin by transmitting forces away from the enthesis (where the tendon attaches to bone). This can usefully allow people to continue to work. If these measures are not sufficient, local injection of hydrocortisone is very useful in diminishing and treating symptoms. Hydrocortisone alone should be used in preference to fluorinated corticosteroids, as the latter may cause atrophy of subcutaneous fat and local disfigurement.

Carpal tunnel syndrome

Carpal tunnel syndrome is due to entrapment of the median nerve as it passes through the carpal tunnel under the flexor retinaculum at the wrist. It is usually idiopathic and may be associated with expansion of the long flexor tendons, but may occur secondarily to other conditions. The causes are:

- Fluid retention—pregnancy or oral contraceptive being the commonest causes.
- Osteoarthritis or rheumatoid arthritis of the wrist
- Colles and scaphoid bone fractures.
- Direct trauma.
- Hypothyroidism.
- Acromegaly.
- Amyloidosis.
- Scheie's syndrome.
- Myelomatosis.

Diagnosis

The diagnosis is made by examination and confirmed by a positive Tinel's sign where percussion of the nerve at the wrist produces pain and para-esthesiae in the median nerve territory. A similar result may also be achieved by sustained full flexion or extension of the wrist (Phalen's sign). Nerve conduction studies and electromyography of the abductor pollicis brevis muscle give the diagnosis and locates the site of the median nerve compression.

Mild carpal tunnel syndrome

- Features:
  - Pain and paraesthesiae occurring in the territory of the median nerve (i.e. the radial aspect of the palmar surface of the hand to include the lateral three and a half fingers).
  - Nocturnal pain causing patients to wake and gain relief by hanging their hand out of bed (cools the limb and reduces symptoms).
- Treatment:
  - Resting the wrist in a volar splint to prevent excessive extension and flexion.
  - Local hydrocortisone injections indicated if splinting alone insufficient.

More severe carpal tunnel syndrome

- Features: motor involvement occurs with abductor pollicis brevis weakness & atrophy.
- Treatment: decompression of the carpal tunnel (particularly where active denervation is present) by removal of a strip of the flexor retinaculum. This has a good prognosis.

De Quervain's stenosing tenosynovitis

Characterized by pain and tenderness on the radial aspect of the wrist due to inflammation of abductor pollicis longus and extensor pollicis brevis tendon sheaths. Occupational activity is often responsible and a positive Finkelstein's test is indicative. This is carried out by flexion and opposition of the thumb into the palm of the hand and held down by the fingers. The wrist is then subjected to an ulnar deviation force, thus stretching the affected tendons and producing pain. Treatment is again through local injection of hydrocortisone, although physical measures can be successful. Addressing the (occupational) cause is important and protecting the wrist in a Futuro™ wrist splint may occasionally be helpful in the short term.

Work-related upper limb disorders

This has commonly been known as the repetitive strain disorder (RSD). Although acute syndromes occur in the workplace, which settle on cessation of the activity, progression to a chronic regional pain syndrome is unclear.

Definition

A number of well-recognized musculoskeletal conditions of the workplace, which is associated with acute, cumulative and chronic 'injuries' and illnesses of soft tissue caused by mechanical stress, strain, sprain and vibration, inflammation or irritation.

Epidemiology

The following points should be noted:
- Women are more affected than men.
- Rare in self-employed people.
- More common in those with mundane repetitive jobs with little job satisfaction.
- Epidemic phenomena are produced in companies or even in a country by the publicity surrounding several cases in which awards were made for compensation.
- Claims can continue to rise despite improvements in working practices.
- Numbers of soft tissue problems fell dramatically when new legislation was introduced to reduce the number of dubious claims.
- Companies with Australian and European offices noted that the problem was more prevalent among Australian employees, despite the fact that all were using the same equipment.
- There was a higher incidence in seasonal workers, such as fruit pickers, just before the end of the season and just before the start of their children's school holidays.
- More common among public sector employees and in those companies whose volume of work was decreasing.
- Symptoms characteristically appear through an increased working demand or a change in practice.

Diagnostic criteria

The clinical diagnosis is made by a history and findings of:
- Upper limb pain in someone whose occupation demands regular and repetitive arm activity.
- Wrist or hand—or less commonly elbow or shoulder—pain.
- Usually starts as limb discomfort accompanied by weakness.
- Leads on to localized tenderness at a tendon/nerve/enthesis in the wrist, forearm, or hand.
- Pain is more commonly confined to the extensor aspect of the limb.
- A common feature is hypersensitivity of overlying structures.
- Decreased pinch grip is the essential factor and a 20% difference between hands is significant.
- If symptoms are bilateral, a 20 Newton decrease (measured by a hand-held dynamometer) from that expected in the normal population is significant.

- Decreased fingertip sensitivity to vibration differentiates between those with genuine pain and those with functional symptoms. A 256 Hz middle C tuning fork on the index and middle fingers gave only 18% false positives and negatives.

The typical patient is a young or middle-aged woman with a long history of arthralgia or myalgia, prolonged morning stiffness, chronic sleep disturbance, and easy fatigue and poor exercise tolerance. She may have other unrelated tender points and acrocyanosis, and there is often subjective swelling of the hands along with non-dermatomal paraesthesiae (pins and needles in a limb, outside a nerve root territory). On examination a degree of dermatographia and considerable impairment of function are present. Pain is often present on moving the neck, but the range of movement is invariably normal. Despite pain-induced muscle power testing, neurological examination is essentially normal. There is a higher prevalence of smoking among sufferers than in the normal female population, but epidemiological studies have not matched subjects for age and social class, which may thus nullify this difference.

Differential diagnosis
- Carpal tunnel syndrome.
- De Quervain's tenosynovitis.
- Lateral or medial humeral epicondylitis.
- Anterior and posterior tibial interosseous syndromes.
- Rotator cuff problems at the shoulder.

Investigations
The diagnosis is clinical and investigations should be kept to a minimum in RSD.

Amputation

Epidemiology

Peripheral vascular disease, the major cause of amputation in the UK, is due to:

- Arteriosclerosis: hypertension, obesity, diabetes itself, hyperlipidaemiam, and smoking.
- Diabetes mellitus: end-stage obliterative arterial, micro-angiopathic, and neurological disease.

Five thousand patients are referred annually for prosthetic treatment (10 000 amputations) (Table 28.1). Upper limb amputation accounts for about 10%. Amputations from trauma and congenital limb deficiency are uncommon, but young users will need an artificial limb for longer and may have more demanding expectations to allow them to return to an active life. Regular limb changes will be required as often as every few months during growth spurts in children.

Table 28.1 UK amputations by age and cause

Aetiology	Age (yr) 0–9	10–19	29–39	40–59	60–79	80+
Trauma	1	33	158	93	41	7
Vascular	2	0	17	294	1563	323
Diabetes	2	0	5	140	507	68
Infection	1	0	13	13	28	2
Malignancy	0	11	26	28	37	10

Planning an amputation

The amputee care team should begin the rehabilitation process as soon as amputation is considered and acts through patient education, defining expectations and artificial limb fitting, as well as advising the surgeon on the choice of surgical operation and the suitability of patients for using artificial limbs. The team also helps and supports patients in the long term.

Information is the key to success, particularly on what it is like to be an amputee, of phantom limb pain and sensation, and stump care. Phantom limb pain is associated with pre-operative pain, and can be reduced by sustained pain relief for at least 72 h before surgery and 48 h afterwards.

Amputation care
- Fitness training: to allow optimal walking, transfers, and standing for long periods.
- Care of the surviving limb is vital, therefore avoid hopping and jumping.
- Amputation level: critical for the expected level of independence, e.g. transtibial and transfemoral, transradial and transhumeral, knee disarticulation.
- Preservation of knee function is the key to independence, it eases transfers and energy of walking and preserves cosmesis.
- Increased energy costs: for above and below knee amputees (as a result of vascular disease) energy costs are increased by 120% and 55% respectively. In bilateral above knee amputees the increase is 280%.
- Prediction of walking: fitness, indication for surgery, age, stump health and length, energy costs, complications.

The limb fitting process

A temporary limb can be fitted within 10 to 14 days after surgery. The post-amputation mobility aid (PPAM) can be fitted as early as 3 to 4 weeks and allows compression of the stump through its air cells (thereby reducing oedema and promoting healing) and early standing, which is useful in the elderly.

Prosthetic treatment

Stump casting and measurement and limb prescription can be done from the 21st post-operative day. Modular systems are used from the very first prescription and temporary cosmetic covers shorten delivery times. Gait re-education with the first prosthesis follows a common sequence:

- Full weight-bearing and weight transfer.
- Walking within parallel bars, turning by stepping.
- Walking with sticks between two parallel bars.
- Walking with one stick between parallel bars.
- Walking with aids out of the bars.
- Optimal gait with minimal walking aids.

The prescription of a prosthesis has to account for the following common features, which interface with the residual limb:

- Socket structure—skeletal structure.
- Articular structures—terminal structures.
- A cosmetic covering—a suspension.

Modern prostheses incorporate design features to improve the gait cycle. The use of intelligent knees and ankle shock absorption allow a smoother gait, reduces energy costs, and resists the forces transmitted during stance and gait without serious risk of mechanical failure. Functional limb prostheses may be body powered, and electronically powered features are now becoming more commonly available. A variety of silicones are used in suction and adhesion devices at the interface, but stump sheaths, called stump socks, are the commonest interface, as they provide considerable relief from shear forces.

A prosthesis has to allow sufficient height for the foot to swing through during the swing phase of the gait cycle. Therefore, heel strike at the start of the next stance phase has to be controlled very quickly, if the artificial leg is to cope with walking forces and the patient has to have the ability to achieve the correct posture and position.

Special needs

Young people with limb deficiency, particularly those with an interest in sport, require robust tensile artificial limbs with adjustable qualities and strong components, e.g. hydraulic swing-phase controls and energy storing and reducing shin/ankle/foot systems. Sleeves are therefore used over the prosthesis for protection, as both exo- and endoskeletal prostheses are not usually waterproof and can prove somewhat hazardous if they get wet.

Outcomes

As in many aspects of disability, it is difficult to find a useful, easily applicable measure of progress during rehabilitation. The Harold Wood/Stanmore Scale and the Guy Scales measure mobility and are currently used in the UK. A Grise Scale is validated as a general outcome measure for amputees, but unfortunately is insensitive to change and it is this very element on which one wishes to gain most information.

Therefore, standard rehabilitation outcome measures are relevant to interventions for amputees and measures of mobility, impairment, activity, and participation/quality of life are used.

Suggested further reading

1 Amputee Medical Rehabilitation Society (1992). *Amputee Rehabilitation. Recommended Standards and Guidelines*. A Report by a Working Party of the AMRS, London. (Copies from AMRS Secretary C/o Royal College of Physicians, 11 St Andrews Place, Regents Park, London NW1 4LE, UK.)

Ageing and disability

Two aspects of ageing need to be considered in physically disabled people: the impact of the ageing process on disabled people and the impact of the disability on the ageing process.

Effect of age on disability

Because of the population's increasing longevity, there is greater pressure on NHS facilities and on the need for care and intermittent rehabilitation.

Effect of disability on age

Are there any differences between the ageing process in disabled and able-bodied individuals? The answer is probably no, but there are specific features which seem to occur more readily in disabled people. The most common aspect of the ageing process in physically disabled people is the appearance of degenerative joint disease, particularly in an increased prevalence of shoulder, hip, and knee osteoarthritis (Fig. 29.1). Radiological changes occur in 54% of men and 58% of women. Joint pain and soreness has also been reported and decreased strength and energy levels are noted, particularly in tetraplegics.

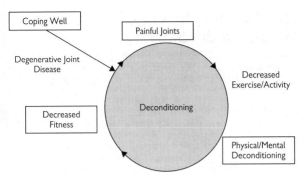

Fig. 29.1 Deconditioning.

Specific examples of ageing features in disability

There are a few classic examples of the effects of ageing in people with long-standing disabilities. The most obvious is the increasing number of co-morbidities leading to difficulties in concentrating on the rehabilitation process.

Spinal injuries

The effects of ageing in spinal cord injury are now being seen, as patients survive with tetra- and paraplegias. Shoulder and neck problems appear to be evident from years of wheelchair propulsion and from the effect of using the upper limbs as weight-bearing structures. A significant proportion require surgery to correct rotator cuff lesions and there is an increased incidence of pressure sores with increasing age. Cardiopulmonary impairments develop and are evident with impaired circulation in the legs and hypertension in tetraplegics. Paraplegics have a profile consistent with the general population. Mortality increases exponentially with age, but there is an extra mortality due to spinal cord injury. However, the mortality ratio decreases with age. Whereas a 20-year-old with a spinal cord injury has a mortality eight times higher than the general population, survivors aged 70 years have a mortality rate of only one and a half times higher. It had been reported that the causes of death mirror the general population and that there is an association with renal failure, particularly again in tetraplegics. However, over the years, since these studies have become more widely known, renal problems have been better addressed and the mortality is much more akin to that of the non-disabled population.

Mobility

The normal ageing process changes one's gait throughout life. As one passes from an infant's gait, which is wide-based and involves pelvic rotation, myelination allows better neuromuscular transmission and growth of bones allows an adult-type gait at around the fifth birthday. Serially, as one gets older, balance mechanisms become less efficient and one naturally shortens the stride length in walking and increases the proportion of the stance phase during the gait cycle during the seventh decade of life. This ensures better stability while walking, but results in decreased walking speed and shortened strides. Increased loading of joints leads to degenerative change in the hip and knee. Similarly, the vectors of the forces coming up the lower limb during this altered gait cycle lead to mild flexion of the trunk, which over years, gives the stooped posture of elderly people. This puts increasing pressure on the articulating facet joints in the lumbar spine, and hence the stiffness and discomfort that can develop.

Traumatic brain injury

There are two age-related peaks in the incidence of traumatic brain injury. In the young, injuries occur from car accidents, etc., but in the elderly they are often due to falls within the home. With multisystem failure, mobility and stability decrease and elderly people fall over more readily. This results in a higher incidence of head injuries and is a reflection more of social and health status rather than the epidemic seen in younger people. However, as with the young, physical and cognitive changes occur to an already failing brain and there is a significant morbidity and mortality attached to traumatic brain injury in the elderly. Additionally, less force is required to damage the skull bones, but elderly people somewhat paradoxically appear to recover better than expected both cognitively and physically after traumatic brain injury.

Post-polio syndrome

This syndrome is classically seen 20 or so years after the development of poliomyelitis-related disability (see Chapter 23). People with poliomyelitis learn to cope with their disability while young, but after a while they notice increasing difficulty carrying out tasks which were previously straightforward, and further investigation shows denervation in the muscles supplied by the affected anterior horn cells. In simplistic terms, it would appear that their lower motor neurones 'burn out' after years of 'overwork' and this possibly represents the effect of normal ageing on a depleted population of anterior horn cells, which have had to supply an expanded number of motor units. There is no evidence that this syndrome has been caused by an awakening of any viral activity in the disease.

Summary

There is an increased incidence in musculoskeletal disease, in strokes, in neurodegenerative disease, and in cancers with increasing age. As stated earlier, the rehabilitation of older people is complicated by the presence of co-morbidities, which slow the rehabilitation process down, and is one of the major differences between rehabilitating the elderly population and a younger disabled population. The needs of both populations are similar in severe disability, as is the impact of the disability. However, there are distinct differences between the support available, the expectations of the individuals compared with the younger population, and very often the aims of rehabilitation. The OPCS survey in 1988 showed that 32% of people with disabilities living in private households were aged 75 years and over, 26% were between the ages of 65 and 64 and 19% between the ages of 55 and 64.

Index